The Bridge

A Seven-Stage Map to Redefine Your Life and Purpose

by Marilyn Powers, Ph.D.
and Steve Viglione

Cover design by Mauricio Hoffman
Edited by Erin-Mari Kelsey
Pre-Press Preparation by Wendy Garrido

The I AM Foundation
7825 Fay Ave Ste 200
La Jolla CA 92037
(619) 297-7010
www.iamfoundation.org

ISBN-10: 9645224-5-4
ISBN-13: 9780964522459

First Published 1999
Revised Edition Published 10/10/2011

Printed in the United States

This book is
a gift from The I AM Foundation,
and Unity Worldwide Ministries.
www.unity.org

Dedication

This book is dedicated to all of you passionate people who choose to take an active role in our worldwide awakening and transformation.

Acknowledgements By Dr. Marilyn Powers

I wish to acknowledge my husband Steve Viglione, Founder and CEO of The I AM Foundation, who gave me the gift of living my mission and purpose. He invited me to be the Co-Founder of The I AM Foundation and to make a significant global impact together. The work we do empowers children and adults to discover their value and bring their value to the world.

I wish to acknowledge Ingrid and Rebekka, my twin daughters, who have been my greatest teachers about unconditional love and having compassion for myself and others.

And to my parents Ruth and Paul, who gave me my first curriculum and set in motion the cycle for my healing and growth.

I wish to acknowledge my relationship to Catherine Ponder, whose teachings on the mental laws of prosperity dramatically affected my life. Without integrating her teachings, I could not have accomplished all that I have today.

And last, but not least, thank you to all the hundreds of clients who have shared their journeys with me and thus were the greatest teachers for my own transformation.

Preface to the Revised Edition

Originally, when I wrote *The Bridge*, I was at a point where many people are getting ready to retire, but I knew retirement wasn't an option. I had fire in my belly. I wasn't "over the hill." I needed a new vision. I needed to expand my purpose. I needed to map out where I had come from, where I was, and most importantly, to figure out where I was going.

And I wasn't alone.

Tens of millions of people like myself were approaching The Bridge. Like me, they couldn't go back to the old ways of living, and yet they had no vision for the future that inspired them. They needed a way to break free of old ways of thinking and of viewing themselves and the world. They needed a new map to travel, a new trip ticket, a new way of being and expressing themselves. They needed a renewal of passion and purpose for their life and future.

At that time, *The Bridge* provided a map for creating an inspiring future.

Twelve years later, in 2010, life is speeding up in all ways. We are confronted by enormous change, both personally and collectively.

A spiritual frame of reference to address the issues that affect us all is more important now than ever.

Already, many of us are frustrated with outside circumstances, which demand that we achieve a psychological and spiritual mastery to effectively respond to the overwhelming amount of change. It is imperative that we seize this moment and view each decade as an opportunity to expand our consciousness and grow.

The healing and growth that in the past could take decades must now be healed and resolved much more quickly.

When the heart is open, everything is possible. When the heart is open, healing and transformation is possible.

Now *The Bridge* is being offered to personally prepare for a great world transition. We are approaching the beginning of a new five thousand year cycle. The Mayans, the Hindus, the Aztecs, and the Hopis all have spoken of the beginning of a new age arising during the winter solstice in the year 2012.

Our personal healing and transformation is necessary for us to create a positive and sustainable future. *The Bridge* offers a Seven-Stage Map to accomplish this endeavor.

It begins with redefining our purpose and life. Instead of being victims of circumstance, we affirm our power to forgive…

"I AM Forgiveness." Instead of self-loathing and deprecation, we affirm what is good and right about us…"I AM Love." And, instead of expressing lack and limitation, we affirm…"I AM Abundance."

Furthermore, we are being called to redefine our mission and purpose, to let go of what no longer serves us and affirm: "Letting go is gain, not loss."

We are being called to embrace the fullness of who we are and to ask the question, "What would I do today if I were brave?" Finally, we are being called to co-create a positive future and a world that serves us all, affirming…"We are One."

Table of Contents

STAGE 4

Bridging the Gap Between Past & Future 133

In this stage, we cover A Major Life Review, Embracing Your Shadow, Letting Go of What No Longer Serves You, and Taking the Best from the Past.

STAGE 5

The Heart of the Journey—Discovering Your Life Purpose & Plan 163

In this stage, we cover Shifting from Personality to Soul, From "What's in it for Me?" To "What Serves Us All?" and Your Mission and Making a Positive Difference in the World.

STAGE 6

Seeking Answers to Life's Ultimate Questions.......... 185

In this stage, we cover Facing Your Mortality, Awakening The Inner Philosopher, Developing Continuity of Consciousness, and Meditation and Lucid Dreaming.

STAGE 7

Coming Home—Union with Source.......................... 215

In this stage, we cover Awakening Your Global Consciousness, Accessing Your Inner Guidance System, and Attracting Your "Soul Group" for Co-creating In Community.

Introduction

Life is a Spiritual Journey

Whether you have been aware of it or not, your life is a spiritual journey, a journey of the soul. The word "spiritual" is often used in confusing ways. All of life—the physical, the emotional, the mental—is spiritual. The spiritual is not something apart from life on earth, but it is essential, fundamental and integral to it. Spirit is not something to be aspired to, for it is already present at every moment. We are simply being called to become aware that everything is spiritual.

Your life can be viewed as a spiritual journey. That is, your experience on this earth is best understood as a journey of the soul. While both your origin and your ultimate destination may remain unknown to you, you will discover that during the time between birth and death, your soul can make a journey of self-evolution—one of healing, growing and transforming. What's more, your soul's journey has distinct stages that correspond (albeit only approximately) to chronological phases of your life. I am inviting you to consciously participate in the spiritual journey of your life.

How many of us have complained that our lives do not come with an instruction manual or that we have never had a map to guide us on our journey? Actually, there have been many early versions of instruction manuals and maps, usually handed down to us in the form of religious instruction or cultural imperatives. These guidelines were imposed on us from the outside, often seen as attempts to mold us and shape us into good citizens and productive members of society.

We are part of a generation of people who have been searching for guidance and direction that comes from deep inside. As part of our process, we have chosen to find our own way whenever possible. At times, we may have temporarily lost our way, or we may have even given up hope of ever finding our way, settling instead for the soul-crushing task of somehow simply surviving. Fortunately, this compromise is no longer necessary or appropriate.

I am communicating to you from a very particular perspective. From this vantage point, I speak compassionately and urgently. A fundamental premise of this book is that there is an underlying design to your soul's journey. In other words, there is a natural process of learning and growth and evolution in the course of your life, which you can learn and master. Some call this process awakening, unfolding, or even enlightenment.

The challenge for most of us has been that we simply have not known that there is such a natural process, much less what it looks like. And as is so often the case with human beings, our ignorance tends to get us into trouble. The good news is that you can now learn to go through this natural process with full awareness. With this view—map and compass in hand—you can consciously make the soul's journey: healing and growing and evolving intentionally.

No matter where you are in your soul's journey, no matter what has happened to you, I know one thing that is true about you: every breath, every action, every experience, every moment of your life has had a meaning and a purpose. Your life is moving forward organically, stage by stage, unfolding as part of an overarching Plan. Nothing has been in vain. You have successfully completed your life's curriculum so far, no matter what "grade" you got.

Your soul's true journey begins with the realization that you are totally responsible for your life on this earth. You are responsible for giving to yourself what wasn't given to you. You are responsible for your growth and evolution. You are responsible for waking up from unconscious living to conscious life. Assistance and support are abundantly available throughout your soul's journey, but you are responsible for creating and attracting the people and circumstances in your life that can support you and help you along the way.

You are also responsible for understanding and mastering the stages of your soul's journey. In this book, you will discover that there is, in your soul's journey, a natural progression, a discernible movement or passage from one stage to another. As you will see, what moves you forward from stage to stage is following your passion. What you are passionate about is the "magnetic North" by which you will learn to set your compass.

Overview of Your Soul's Journey

This is my view of the soul's journey via a seven-stage map that I want to share with you:

Stage 1: Enlightenment Through Pain

Your journey begins as a response to *pain*: when you admit that the inevitable *life pain* you are experiencing is unacceptable or intolerable, and you actively *seek and find help*. This reaching out puts your foot on the path, so to speak. This begins *enlightenment through pain.*

Stage 2: Developing a Positive Self-Concept

You begin developing the capacity to love and accept yourself unconditionally. This ushers in the birth of an appropriate and stable *self-concept*.

Stage 3: Having What You Want

Grounded in yourself, you develop the mental skill of *manifestation*, creating an abundance of *goodness* in your life—a sustainable balance of health, love, well-being, material support and financial independence.

Stage 4: The Bridge, i.e., The Impasse Between Past & Future

At every major change, you are faced with aspects of yourself that you have ignored or suppressed. Your *Shadow*—the unconscious and unexpressed parts of yourself—makes itself known. As you learn to integrate this shadow-self, it alters your life, often in unexpected ways. This part of the journey is a time of re-evaluating and re-examining what to keep and what to let go.

Stage 5: Discovering Your Life Purpose and Plan

Now you begin discovering your life's purpose and plan, and move to accomplish your unique mission on this earth. As you do so, you learn how your life plan fits into the whole of humanity. You begin doing *world work*.

Stage 6: Seeking Answers to Life's Ultimate Questions

At this stage, you are confronted by the reality that your physical life will end—and, at the same time, you discover experientially that you are more than your body, your thoughts and your emotions. In other words, you become aware of both your mortality and your immortality. Your self-concept expands, giving way to a connection with the Self.

Stage 7: Coming Home—Union with Source

At last, you enter into a state of Oneness, a world without separation, a life without polarity, a realm of Union with the Source of all Creation. Here, your life is focused on co-creating the future.

The Two Curriculums

The Bridge speaks about two curriculums...

The First Curriculum

The first curriculum we receive at birth from our parents, family of origin, education, culture and religion. Before we took our first breath, took our first step, our whole life was planned out for us. All the scripts and programs, the expectations were laid out for us.

Some of us may have rebelled, resisted, fought the curriculum. Others may have made compromises; they have sacrificed what they genuinely wanted for what they thought was expected or approved of. And some may have followed the program and done a "good job." Nevertheless, whether you liked it or not, the first curriculum was a given.

The Second Curriculum

The second curriculum, however, is very different. It has not been formulated and still needs to be designed. Unlike the first, we cannot look back to past generations and traditions. It won't come from outside sources like social systems and culture. The foundation of this curriculum is within us. It originates from our healing and the transformation of our personal and collective psyche.

Here, your course of learning can go far beyond survival and meeting your personal needs. The second curriculum opens the way to an expansion of the self, based on an understanding of the underlying design of your soul's journey. This part of the journey will find you confronting your mortality as well as the question of what happens after death. Focusing on your life purpose, you will find the opportunity to engage in the planetary community and participate in a larger purpose.

Mastering the Seven Stages

"Enlightenment" is often seen as a state to be achieved, the goal of the soul's journey. However, such goal-oriented striving for a state of consciousness is often undertaken at stages where one is inadequately equipped for the task. One cannot proceed directly from being a toddler learning how to walk to being a fully enlightened master. There is a lot of growing and developing that must occur along the way. The focus *here* is on the process of growing up, not so much on what it's like when we finally get there.

Part of my intention in this book is to offer some practical guidelines for avoiding the swamps and distractions of the stages of the journey, as well as what to do when you find yourself up to your armpits in alligators. As you explore this map to the seven stages of your soul's journey, there are several general principles or guidelines that are worth keeping in mind:

1. Not everyone goes through all seven stages of the journey in a single lifetime.

2. The process is very forgiving. Mistakes and poor choices can be worked through. After all, as you will discover, you are here *to learn and grow*, not to be perfect. The object is not to "get it right," but to *complete the work you have to do.*

3. The journey requires your active, conscious effort. There is no way to make the journey of the soul *passively.*

4. It is likely that your progress will not always be straightforward. For instance, reaching an impasse (a *Stage Four* phenomenon) could plunge you back into Enlightenment through Pain. Or you could stall for a long time in the swamp of attachment to materiality in *Stage Three.* A sudden brush with death (*Stage Six*) could easily bring up unfinished business from life's first curriculum. Or achieving a high degree of financial success without having worked through self-concept issues (*Stage Two*) could lead you to a painful *starting over.*

5. You do not have to die or get a new body to start a new curriculum.

6. Growing into your "*Self*" means letting go of attachment to your separate self. This requires practice and inner discipline.

7. You need not consider anything to be *true* (including what is said in this book) until it is part of your *personal experience*.

8. You cannot make the soul's journey alone. *We are in this together.*

Purpose

This book is a guide for self-exploration and discovery, for learning and unfolding. It will provide you a larger context, a perspective from which you can view the spiritual adventure of life. I am offering you a clear map of your soul's journey between the time of birth and death, as well as a compass to assist you in understanding the stage which you are currently moving through. Here you will gain practical insight into the challenges and rewards of each stage of the journey, plus some simple but powerful tools that you may find helpful along your way.

The Bridge is part of a great awakening. This book is intended to inspire a movement of passionate people who choose to take an active role in this worldwide transition and awakening. Out of this movement are emerging *soul groups*, people who find themselves in deep alignment and resonance with each other, sharing a purpose of co-creating a planetary future based on the wisdom of love, not fear. Linked through electronic and empathic communication, anchored in international physical centers that serve as hubs and gathering points, all guided by a 21st century *school for conscious evolution*, we are building a global virtual community of co-creators—together.

--*Dr. Marilyn Powers*
Sonoma, California, 2011

Stage 1

Enlightenment Through Pain

Pain is a pathway to awareness.

In this stage, we cover Honoring Your Pain, Letting Go of The Museum of Resentments and Regrets, and Creating the Parent You Never Had.

How You Got Here

You enter this life unaware. As a newborn infant, you do not know who you are or why you are here or what life is all about. You receive your first information about yourself and the world through and from your biological parents. From them, you receive your physical and emotional makeup, your outlook on life, your most basic feelings about yourself.

As you grow up, you are programmed and conditioned—first by your family of origin and then by the community that brought you up.

Television may play a major role in the shaping of your consciousness. Your religious upbringing could also be a significant factor. You are further influenced—although perhaps not as much—by the educational institutions that seek to guide you.

Enlightenment through pain is an inner, organic process where you will be submerged in all of your feelings—your helplessness, your rage, your weeping, your jealousy.

Your total environment, your culture, your society, the world you grow up in, and your experiences—plus your own thoughts, feelings, beliefs and reactions—all play a part in forming your concept of yourself and your world. From this milieu, you develop a number of "scripts," or unconscious patterns of behavior that are triggered *automatically* by your perceptions of what is happening around you. Unknown to you, these scripts largely dominate your life, determining your choices and actions in ways of which you are scarcely aware. *And, unbeknownst to you, these same scripts determine how you perceive yourself.*

Your scripts guide you through *life's first curriculum*. You know that you are supposed to grow up, get yourself educated, develop your body and your mind, choose a career, find love, get married, have a family, and build yourself a reasonably secure foundation for the future. This is the curriculum that you are given from the moment of birth, and you spend the first part of your life doing your best to master it. Like a lot of people, you may be able to live this way for quite a long time, acting out the pre-programmed scripts of your first curriculum. In fact, many people go to their deathbeds without realizing there is more to life. No, not you. You are determined to have your life be more than that.

Depending on your lot in life, your conditioning probably does a fairly good job in propelling you to create the kind of life you believe you should have—up to a certain point. On the other hand, having what you want in life might seem difficult and endlessly frustrating.

In either case, sooner or later, things no longer seem to work for you. You become dissatisfied with the life you are living, or you may experience feelings of ennui, boredom, numbness, depression or free-floating anxiety. A fog may seem to settle into your life.

Perhaps you experience a breakdown in your primary relationship – a divorce or a painful affair. Perhaps your career suddenly goes awry. Your company downsizes, and you are out of work. Or you find you can simply no longer take punching the time clock day after day. You might even try going into business for yourself, only to find that it is much harder than you thought. Nothing seems to work anymore.

Regardless of how it begins for you, at some point, your life becomes intolerable. You find that your life is characterized by unrelenting *pain* – mental, emotional, and perhaps even physical (illnesses have an uncanny tendency to show up at this point). You may notice that you're under a lot of *stress*. For a time, you may try various ways of avoiding or minimizing the pain, such as alcohol, drugs, sex, or even burying yourself in your work. But these strategies always backfire. Eventually, the pain resurfaces, each time becoming more difficult to deal with.

By now, you are getting desperate. More than anything else, you want things to *change*. You want your life to be different. You don't want to experience this pain any more. You admit to yourself that avoiding the pain is no longer possible. You're ready to do *anything* to have things be different in your life, but you don't know what to do. You simply don't know how to get out of the pain.

Marty and Cindy attended an experiential workshop—their stories illustrate how pain ruled their life. Marty was a 38-year-old doctor—handsome, silent, shut down, married with three young kids and afraid to communicate. He was out of touch with his feelings, afraid to speak up and didn't have the foggiest idea of what he would want to communicate about himself. There was a deep void inside him. He didn't know what he believed or thought, and to him feeling was out of the question. He was totally unable to tap into his emotions except for the most fundamental needs. He was lonely and without a single close friend. When his wife complained—he withdrew physically and emotionally. She would then mirror his depression. His external mask of success had worn thin—inside he was terrified and unable to connect to anything or anyone outside his role of doctor.

Cindy, on the other hand, had been separated from her husband for nine months—after being married for 18 years. Her husband, twice her age, was verbally abusive and emotionally controlling. Cindy now lived alone with her two sons who were eight and ten years old. She believed she wanted her independence, although she was terrified and overwhelmed at the thought of being on her own. She found herself waking up in the middle of the night unable to sleep, vacillating back and forth as to whether she should go back to what was familiar or go forward into the unknown. She was frozen in fear and feeling incapable of making decisions. Even though she sought autonomy, she was still financially and emotionally dependent on a "father-figure" as a caretaker and provider.

If this sounds or feels familiar—welcome to the first stage of the journey, the time of *enlightenment through pain*. [1]

The Lay of the Land

If this is where you find yourself, the pain you have been experiencing is a signal that something is wrong. This pain has been trying to get your attention for a long time. It might help to know there is finally nothing to do but face the pain, and learn how to change yourself. For so long you have been unconscious, running on automatic. This is the time for waking up.

Why are a lot of people depressed? Because they have a lot of unhappiness inside them, and they don't want to face it. They're looking for an immediate remedy—for example, by getting on anti-depressants. They don't know how to access their feelings in a controlled or helpful way. Why do some people seem one-dimensional and shallow? It's not because they're shallow, but because everything is underground. There is so little that they know about who they are beyond the social and professional definition, or their parental scripts. As with Marty, the one and only place in his life that he felt safe, good about himself and able to positively connect to people was in his helping role as a physician. Outside of that professional context he was unable to effectively interact and communicate.

The Symptoms

If your journey has taken you to *enlightenment through pain*, you are experiencing a lot of turmoil in your life. Things seem to be spinning out of control. You feel hopeless, or helpless, experiencing bouts of depression. Or you're just downright unhappy. Most of the time you feel numb, without a lot of emotion or feeling. You appear tepid, neutral, bored. When you do express your emotions, they are mostly irritability, impatience or anger. Or you have *no* emotions, and your affect is flat. You're dull. There's no energy or excitement in your life. You're not living in the present, but constantly seeing things through the lens of the past.

Chaos and confusion reign in your relationships, at home and at work. You encounter a lot of fighting, projecting, blaming, criticizing, and judging. Trust is often a major issue. You keep running into control issues—your own, and others'. In general, you feel very disconnected from people. Even though you attempt to seek out people who think exactly the way you do, you usually feel separate and alone. If you're still in a marriage, you feel like you're just going through the motions, the rituals. Emotionally, you're in struggle and disharmony. You may be going through a divorce. It seems that you keep cycling through the same painful patterns in your intimate or family relationships.

Facing the prospect of dealing with all the pain, anxiety, fear and helplessness alone, you may feel almost overwhelmed. You feel like a victim of circumstance, with a lot of rage and blame: *How can this be happening to me? How could they do this to me?* It's bad enough that *you* are suffering, but much to your horror you discover that you also *cause* suffering in the lives of others. It seems that you are no longer in charge of your life. "Doing the right thing" doesn't seem to get you where you want to go any more. Your old ways of getting things done, where you always knew what to do, don't work anymore. Life has become a struggle. You're not "successful," in your own terms. At the same time you feel very dependent on the systems around you (family, work, and community) and you resent it. Real security seems beyond your reach. You experience anxious, sleepless nights or panic attacks.

Your programming, filters, and beliefs are all based on past scripting. It's the scripting of the past that creates pain in the present.

In an effort to cover up the pain, you've developed some serious addictions that are now running you rather than supporting you or making things better. These may include the abuse of medications, coffee, cigarettes, alcohol, drugs, or sex. You might become a "workaholic." Or you may stuff yourself with food. Your rare spare time is spent glued to your armchair in front of the television set, trying not to think about your life.

If this is where you are, you feel like you're stuck in a rut or on a treadmill. You have a gnawing sense deep in your gut that something's wrong or missing in your life. You wonder, *What's the point of it all?*

Guidelines for Enlightenment Through Pain

What You Can Expect

With these painful feelings, going on anti-depressants may be seductively inviting. But in the larger context, this is actually the time when you need to begin to face yourself, re-examine your values and the way you think, and re-think the way you organize your life. The pain is not something to escape from or even put up with. You don't have to believe *this is just the way the world is* or *this is just the way my life is*. What is beckoning to you now is a way to move out of the pain of ignorance and illusion.

In enlightenment through pain, you live 80% of your life in past time. Rarely are you here and now. You're constantly seeing things through the lenses and emotions of the past.

This is the time to connect with a *personal guide*—a teacher, therapist or group who can help you begin to wake up, to change in the ways that will support your growth. It is very important to realize that most people *cannot make this journey alone*. In addition to your guide, you will also need the support of others who are going through the journey themselves.

Enlightenment through pain is often the stage when people look outside for help. Tia, a participant in a group, was a single woman in her mid 30s. She was definitely a professional and financial big hitter. She was, however, going through the third break-up of a five-year relationship. She was at her wits' end being with a man who could not commit to the relationship and who lied to her. She was hurt, confused, and feeling that after three tries she had struck out.

She knew that if she ran her business the way she ran her personal relationship, she would be out on the street penniless. Instead of being financially bankrupt, shelt emotionally bankrupt. She began asking why she allowed herself to be with someone who continually lied to her and let her down. Why couldn't she leave when it seemed obvious that would be the appropriate thing to do? All of her friends supported her leaving but that wasn't enough to help her get out of this dead-end situation. In the group she found she shared similar issues—other women struggling with painful relationships. She realized she was not alone. The women in the group were intelligent and capable and still needed help emotionally. It was part of their journey discovering that they created their pain and that they could somehow change outcomes.

This stage demands tremendous perseverance and compassion. You are going to be doing a lot of re-thinking and re-evaluating of your life. This is a time for self-examination. You will come to see how your conditioning and your "history bank" have blinded you in terms of knowing what's true, and have kept you from finding the point of power inside yourself. You are coming out of numbness and unconsciousness. You must be willing to become aware of your pain, acknowledge it, express it and experience it fully to be conscious. You will become aware of what is going on inside you, giving notice and attention to yourself for perhaps the first time in your life. You will go through an inner and outer dialogue that will move you from darkness to light.

If you are at this point of the journey you have a lot of work to do on yourself. This will be a process and it's going to take some time and effort. Know that you have a lot to learn. You will need to adopt the forgiving, patient attitude of a learner. As you take responsibility for your pain, you will have to learn to forgive yourself and others, release, and let go of the past. You will be taking responsibility for giving yourself everything that you feel you lack.

In reviewing her history with her parents, Tia further realized how much her mother neglected her as a child—to the extreme of not washing her hair for days or not taking her to the dentist for several years. When Tia's dog disappeared, her mother told her it had been run over when, in fact, her mother had given it away. At the same time, her father had violent mood swings and would fly into a rage with little provocation. To protect herself, she avoided all contact with him. At an early age, she discovered that she couldn't depend on either of her parents—that they couldn't make an emotional commitment to her or be trusted to tell her the truth. The only person she could rely on was herself; therefore it wasn't a big surprise to her to be in a relationship that wasn't a whole lot better. Before Tia could attract an appropriate man who would make a commitment to her—she had to make a commitment to herself. This commitment was to draw the people, circumstances and resources that could assist her on her journey. She was no longer alone; she could face the future with an ever-expanding supportive and nurturing network.

Most important, this is the moment you must take responsibility for your life, and *want* to change. *You must commit to your own healing.* This commitment will draw to you the people, circumstances and resources that will assist you on your journey.

Stress and Illness

It is tempting to label what is happening to you as *stress.* You may be saying to yourself, "I'm in a lot of stress because of my job," or "I'm stressed out over my financial situation." But this is just a facade. This is not a matter of stress but a matter of ignorance, of not knowing yourself. You are experiencing a lot of pain simply because you're operating from the misperceptions, misconceptions and illusions of the past. The value of "stress" is that it brings you to want to step on the path to healing. Whether it is physical, emotional or mental stress, it can motivate you to find the *cause* of stress in your life. There are times I call stress a "ketchup" word. Children use excessive ketchup when they don't like the food they have been given. It's a way of covering up what they don't like.

Stress alerts you to look deeper, to see the causes. It's time to bring your life back into balance, to make sense of your life and what you're doing. Stress shows you that you don't know how to access your own wisdom, your inner resources, your higher principles and values. You need a new perspective that can help you understand your past and how it's influencing you now.

This was certainly true of Rob, a corporate president, who joined a men's group after a year of trying to find out the cause of an abnormal swelling in his neck. Although the doctors had no explanation, his neck was one third larger than its normal size. After two months in the group, he realized that his problem was stress-related—primarily because he didn't know how to set boundaries at work. He was incapable of saying no to anyone who wanted to see him. When reviewing his life, he uncovered the source of his problem. His father had died when he was 10 years old, and being the oldest son, Rob became the man of the house. This meant that all of his siblings turned to Rob for advice and support. He was always there and prided himself for never turning anyone away. When he left home and started his own small business, his philosophy was to have an open-door policy. As in his childhood, everyone always had access to him. Several years later, when he sold his successful business, he was hired to run a large corporation. This time, however, it didn't work to have an open-door policy. Now, due to the nature of the corporate culture, he was going to be forced to set boundaries, learn to say no, and delegate more of the responsibility. Within two months of finding out that the script from the past was controlling his choices in the present, he was able to define his boundaries. With this change in attitude, his physical symptoms disappeared. Without those symptoms, however, he would have never been able to get to the source of the problem and thereby affect a more conscious change in his interpersonal behavior at work.

These days, it's not unusual for physical illness to be the first sign of enlightenment through pain – cancer, arthritis, or heart disease. It's no wonder these are known as "stress-related" diseases. There's nothing like a sudden, unexpected heart attack to wake you up.

Oh, I have to eat differently to feel differently. I have to change my diet in order for me not to have certain kinds of symptoms. I begin meditation and deep relaxation as a way of lowering the stress and centering myself.

It is also the time when many suddenly start having inexplicable panic attacks. Actually, these are the lucky ones. Some people manage to remain 30 or 40 years in unconsciousness before they step on the path and look at the journey they've been traveling. A panic attack or illness is a clear signal, a cry for help.

Timing

The time of enlightenment through pain can come at virtually any time in your adult life. It first showed up for me in my late 20s, and it ultimately drove me into therapy – which led to a very rewarding career. On the other hand, many people manage to avoid this inevitable stage for a long time, with their lives seeming to go along just fine, for the most part. But then something happens – a wrenching event that unmasks the pain hidden underneath – and the bottom falls out. For many, this can happen in their 40s or 50s.

In fact, the *mid-life crisis* is usually an experience of being suddenly plunged into enlightenment through pain.

Making Choices

The Decision to Heal

In many ways, Stage One is all about making choices. The first decision you need to make is to change so that you can heal. The "enlightenment" part of enlightenment through pain is that you make a commitment to yourself.

The decision that leads to commitment draws to us the people, situations and circumstances that can help us.

Jay was dealing with being fired for the third time in two years. He couldn't grasp why this kept happening to him. What was wrong with him? Wanting to understand, Jay joined a group and began talking about his childhood. He recalled the competitiveness he had with his father. He described how important it was for his father to be right and always have the last word. Jay would get frustrated when his father rejected his ideas and opinions. It was only after discussing his childhood that he realized that each time he argued with a superior, he was replaying the same interaction that he had with his father as a boy. Now Jay understood that he viewed all his superiors in the same light as his father—and why it was so important for him to have the last word and to be right. Jay not only needed to make the connection with his past, he also needed help in letting go of the need to be right and have the last word. What he genuinely wanted was to be heard and respected even when there was a difference of opinion. It was important for him to learn to accept differences as something to be expected. In fact, he discovered that once he experienced someone truly listening to his point of view, it was easier to accept a difference and not feel compelled to force agreement. With help and practice communicating, Jay was able to hold onto his next job.

You decide that you are going to learn whatever you need to learn, to do whatever it takes, to go through whatever you have to go through – no matter what it costs or how long it takes – in order to heal. You finally arrive at the point where you are compelled to take action:

I'm not going to accept this anymore. I don't know how to change it, but I know I want to change it. I am going to reach out for help in understanding why I am in this predicament of pain. My conditioning probably causes it, by my ignorance and by the curriculum that I've received from my parents and my whole life situation. My conditioning is simply inadequate, full of holes and illusions. I need to learn something about why I'm here and how I created this for myself. I want to find out what it is in me that needs to change in order to experience my life differently. I am ready to change, ready to heal.

I don't want to be numb anymore. I am going to feel the pain. I am going to honor my feelings. I am going to find out what is the source of them. I know the source is in me, in my programming, in my scripts, in my ignorance, in my misperceptions, in my distortion of values. I'm going to learn to understand how I think and feel, and how I can shift and change all of that to affect changes in my life.

Getting Help

The first step in enlightenment through pain is the awareness that *with help,* you can do something about it. Once you have made the decision to change and heal, seeking and finding the help you need is your first priority.

Of course, you can do some things for yourself through reading certain self-help books, reflecting, or going to seminars and workshops. But none of these will substitute for working with someone who can listen to you deeply, who understands the challenges you're facing and knows how to help you find your way. If you have a toothache, you don't just try to stop the pain by yourself. You find a professional you can trust, someone who knows exactly what needs to be done. When the pain is great enough, you will know it's time to find real help.

Perhaps you're the kind of person who believes, *I'm going to take care of myself. I'm the only one I can trust. I'll fix this myself. I'll figure it out. I always did, and I always will.* Know that this attitude is just part of your pain, part of the ignorance, because in reality you're separated and disconnected from people.

If you don't reach out for help now, then you are basically stuck in your own drama. You are unconsciously living out your pain. You are reactive, going into projection and blame. You are being a victim, and you can be in this state of pain and suffering for many years.

You might think at first, *I'm going to change this*. You do everything you can think of, all the ways you've used before, to make it better. But the pain doesn't go away. It re-occurs. You find that no matter what you do, you can't change it. To your dismay, you begin to "stub your own toe" over and over. Your chronic pain may escalate to acute pain, requiring medical attention.

Until you wake up to the fact that you need *help* in dealing with your pain, you are likely to stay stuck in this rut of unconsciousness, unable to break out of your non-productive routines, your self-destructive patterns and your unhappiness. If you continue to "go it alone," you may remain a prisoner of your scripts, your beliefs and your reactions. Your own unconscious programming could keep you blind to other possibilities for change and healing. You may become resentful, or simply give up and shut down.

You need help to get through this. *You didn't get into this situation alone, and you won't be able to get out of it alone.* So you ask yourself, "*Is there a doctor for the soul, someone who can help heal my pain, my unhappiness?*" The answer is yes! There is help available. And you have the inner resources to attract exactly what you need. Once you make the decision to find help, if you persist, you will draw to yourself the assistance you need. *Never give up.*

If you don't reach out for help now, you are basically stuck in your own drama. You are unconsciously living out your pain. You are reactive, going into projection and blame. You are being a victim, and you can be in this state of pain and suffering for many years.

Self-Correction and "Perfection"

Somewhere inside yourself you may be thinking: *Do I really have to go through this? Do I really have to change?* Perhaps you have read, or have been told, that you are "perfect" just the way you are, that everything is perfect, that everything is happening perfectly—just as it should. Yet, this is not what you're *feeling* on the inside. You know that something is not right. No matter how hard you try to believe things are somehow perfect, you just can't do it.

No one is perfect. All of the scripts you learned have holes in them. Therefore you are going to experience pain, and the pain is a signal that you need to self-correct.

Whenever you experience pain, it *is* perfect because the pain is telling you that something is wrong, that you need to self-correct. You are a learner. You have just received a message that you're out of alignment, that you need to change something inside yourself. That's good news, an opportunity to heal something that you may not have been aware of before. And that's perfect.

If you were perfect, you wouldn't need to come to this life. This is a school for learners, not masters. *Enlightenment through pain* is an essential part of being here on the planet. The fact that you are not perfect makes earth the perfect place for you to be. You are perfect for this journey!

Entering into the Spiritual Journey

Enlightenment through pain is a therapeutic, creative process that leads you from the darkness to the light. That's why it's a *journey*—because there's movement *through* the pain. When you see your life as a spiritual journey, then you want to understand your life, the "first curriculum" that you were given at birth. You want to understand your family, your background, and your history. And you want to make the pain a point of enlightenment.

Sometimes people say, "Well, of course, I love myself." But it doesn't have any depth to it. Why? Because the part that they love is the role they perform, the persona they present. Ask them about the other parts of themselves, and they will say, "That's unimportant. That's not really me."

Remember that you are entering into a *process* here. Your healing and transformation will not happen overnight. Patience and perseverance are so important. There are whole parts of yourself that you are just beginning to discover and learn about. In other words, you only know the *tip of your personal iceberg*. In a way, you are like an impenetrable mountain of rock-solid ice. Imagine what would happen if the ice melted all at once and there was a raging flood, completely out of control. That's exactly what nearly all of you fear most—that if you start this process, you'll be overwhelmed and drown. No wonder you hesitate. You don't want to have all your defenses suddenly ripped away.

In a healing context, the melting occurs slowly, gently. With patience and persistence, you become aware of your history—the events and memories that have shaped you—and allow the warmth of the sunlight to gradually dissolve your iceberg into drops of understanding that will eventually flow into a life-giving stream. It's also important to realize that the time of enlightenment through pain marks the initial stages of your soul's journey, because it is the moment you *begin* to awaken and your consciousness begins to unfold. In darkness, you are entering into the tunnel. Eventually, if you persist, you *will* move into the light.

Stage One Work

Okay, you've made the commitment to yourself. You've chosen to learn to get to the roots of your pain and to heal. You've found someone to guide you through the process, a therapist or some wise soul who knows the territory of Stage One. You ask yourself, What's the curriculum here? What will I need to be working on during my passage through enlightenment through pain?

Honoring Your Pain

If you don't feel the pain, you don't know you need to address it. Your pain tells you there is a problem here; therefore, the pain isn't to be ignored or medicated.

The pain you have been experiencing is a mirror of who you are on the inside. You are simply reaping the consequences of your own programming, your conditioning, your unconscious beliefs, and your thoughts. So the first part of the work is to honor your own pain. After all, it is the pain that finally takes you out of unconsciousness and motivates you to wake up. The pain guides you to the places inside yourself where you are not whole, not healed, and not awake.

In recent years, mythologist Joseph Campbell and others have advised that you are to "follow your bliss." This has become deeply embedded in the human potential culture. And that is good advice for some people, if they have already completed their work in Stage One. If, on the other hand, you are dealing with enlightenment through pain issues, it's far better for you to *follow your pain!* Let your pain be your *friend*. So, *follow* your pain to its roots, because it is telling you where the healing in your life needs to take place. As you go through the process of healing, you will wake up to what you need to let go of, release, cleanse and clarify. If you're in pain, all it means is that you're in the dark. You need a way of waking up and understanding the pain, not minimizing it. You will discover that *whatever you unconsciously repress gains energy and power over you*. It becomes your blind spot, the way you always undo your good. Or it becomes the way you resist love and refuse to accept the positive in your life. You can say to yourself:

> *I am going to feel the pain. I will honor these feelings, and I will find their source. Their source is within me, in my programming, in my scripts, in my ignorance, in my misperceptions, in my distorted values. I am going to learn how I think and feel and discover how I can change so that I can effect a change in my life.*

Rediscovering Your Lost Self

In the early phases of Stage One, you work on exploring your personal biography; experiencing your feelings of pain, hurt, disappointment and rage; having compassion for yourself; acknowledging your unmet needs that were unknown to you. You are expanding your awareness of yourself.

Along the way, you will discover and acknowledge the pain of the child you once were, and the child that still lives within you. Kate came to a weekend workshop because she had great difficulty in acknowledging her need for support and help. She grew up with an alcoholic father who physically abused her mother. There were times when he was in a drunken stupor that he would mistake Kate for her mother and lash out at her. To exacerbate the problem, her mother was also an alcoholic who was depressed and passive. She often neglected her children by withdrawing into her bedroom. Over the years, Kate too had isolated herself and focused on controlling her environment, leaving nothing to chance or surprise. Being the second oldest of four children, she felt the burden of responsibility caring for her younger brother and sister. Now, at 34 years old, she was having anxiety attacks when she was asked to leave her position at a law firm where she had made a safe and secure niche for herself. She struggled to find the motivation to overcome her fear of change. As she explored her childhood she started to acknowledge her lost self. She remembered standing between her father and mother trying to protect her mother from being hit by her father. She would hide in a closet for hours, too scared to come out, and went to bed each night gritting her teeth. With no mother to protect her and a father who terrorized her, Kate had lost contact with her inner dependent child very early. As she recalled these events of her childhood, she was able to acknowledge the child's need for protection. Now she could begin to form a relationship to the child within her.

With all of the work that's been done over the years on the inner child, you now know that the child inside contains all your memories. As an adult, you have the opportunity to take your inner emotional child into a therapeutic or healing context. In that safety, your inner child will begin to experience what it's like to have an emotionally nurturing and supportive, wise parent, who wants to hear everything the child has experienced. A parent who wants to understand the pain, who wants to validate and acknowledge everything that has happened to this precious child. Very early on in your life, whole parts of your being were lost because the family into which you were born did not accept them. This is a crucial realization—whole parts of you have been repressed or rejected, denied or minimized. The way you function became limited. You no longer had access to all of who you are. You started making pseudo-adaptations and lost touch with your feelings, to the point that often you really didn't know yourself. You began operating and making decisions with a very small part of yourself.

Listening to the Pain

At this stage, you are honoring your pain. You are feeling your emotions, expressing your grief and your rage. You can no longer rest content in numbness or compulsive doing. You get it touch with your needs and begin expressing them. You *communicate*.

If you allowed yourself to cry and let out all the pain you have inside, would your tears fill a stream? A river? A lake? An ocean? Are you willing to honor your pain and not minimize it?

This is very important to understand in the therapeutic relationship, whether it is with an individual therapist or other healer, or a support group. Most likely, no one really ever listened to you in your family. At this point in your life, being *heard* is an essential part of your healing process. As someone hears you on the outside, you begin to trust and listen to yourself on the inside. You need to know that whenever you express yourself, someone will be there to deeply listen to you, to pay attention to and honor what you're saying. For many of you, this is a first-time experience.

The therapeutic or healing relationship provides you a container where someone really wants to hear you, to feel you, and to be with you in your pain. Someone is there to help you move through your darkness into the light. You can't circumvent the pain. You can't go around it. You must go through it. And part of the process is to expose and disclose what is deep inside, what you have been afraid to express and look at for most of your life.

If you stayed inside the disguise, concealing the pain, you would never be able to feel that anyone truly loves you. You would always suspect that if someone saw this dark side of you, they would not accept you, they could not love you. And if you don't believe that any one could love you if they really knew you, then you cannot truly love yourself—or anyone else, for that matter.

Like most everyone, you've probably been working hard to cover up those hidden parts of yourself with a facade. But it never works for very long. In a therapeutic or healing context, you will tell the whole story, and you will be heard. Someone will be there to say, "Yes, what you have experienced is painful. But together we're going to accept everything that happened as part of your life. We're going to accept you with your weaknesses and your strengths. We're going to accept the whole package." This message marks a major milestone in your soul's journey, the beginning of being able to accept and honor your process.

Your Commitment to Do the Work

Your level of commitment will affect the healing process. You probably have heard stories of people in apparently endless therapy.

You might even know someone going through the process and think, "Well, they've been in therapy for such a long time, but not a whole lot seems to have changed." It may have something to do with their commitment to do the work. You will be drawn to the therapeutic context or therapist or healer or situation that reflects the level of change you want.

First, you become aware of the pain. You reach out for some form of help, and that can come in many different ways—a workshop, a book, a friend, therapy. And at some point, after the initial impulse to change, you realize you need to *commit* to make changes in yourself. And you realize you can't do it by yourself.

Eventually, you find someone who you feel could actually take you through the tunnel. It could be a person, a succession of workshops, a therapy group, an educator, a healer, a class or a school. This is when you believe it can happen that you can begin to work through pain to enlightenment. In reality, you may need a series of situations or people to assist you.

Working on Your Personal History Bank

To know your pain is to know yourself. To know yourself is to come to understand your history bank, your personal biography, the melodrama that has been unfolding in your life. You have to know and honor the scripts and conditioning that have been running you before you can release them. You can't just dispose of them because you don't like them.

Some of the questions that may come up for you are these: Are you one who blames, or are you a victim? Which role have you chosen to play? Do you flip back and forth? Do you prefer to be a victim? Do you prefer to project your anger and hurt? Have you minimized your personal biography? Do you have the attitude that this is all behind you and has no relevance to you today? Or do you recognize you have unfinished business with either or both of your parents, families or siblings? Are you in a power struggle in your primary relationship?

At this point, you have to personally deal with the contents of your life—*all of them*, not just the initial symptoms that woke you up to the pain and told you that you needed help. This means that a therapeutic or healing context is essential. This will be a process of education and learning. In enlightenment through pain, you look at the larger context of your life. You need to understand the beliefs and scripts that have been creating your pain. You have a lot of cleansing and releasing of negativity to do because your vision and perceptions are skewed.

The cause of your pain is that you don't really know how to think correctly. You're a victim of your programming and your belief systems. You're in a circle, and you don't know how to get yourself out. You don't have a point of reference to begin to look at your process, to begin to build the self-acceptance that embraces you where you are on the journey. You need a process of self-discovery to understand how you have created these circumstances and begin to take charge of them.

One of those processes of healing is that you're no longer going to submit and resent. You're going to verbalize what you feel and think. And, yes, you're going to begin to look at the events in your personal history bank and see how they've affected you.

Peter was caught up in a painful relationship with his wife. For years he had been silent and succumbed to it: first numb, then scared, and eventually getting in touch with his resentment. As he began remembering the beatings he received as a child from his father, he also remembered seeing his father fly into a rage when seeing a B on a report card. Peter never quite understood what was so bad about getting a B. This experience taught Peter to fear his father's disapproval and learned to say nothing and to submit. It was then that Peter's will was broken; it was then that he stopped speaking up for himself. Isolated and alone, how could Peter expect to assert himself, ask for his needs to be met, communicate or expect to be heard? Now, in his marriage, he continued the same program he learned in childhood.

Remember that you're going to *re-frame your history*. You came to this planet as a learner, not because you're perfect. Your pain is simply part of the curriculum for your education. Your parents are learners, too. In some way, you contracted with them when you chose to enter your family group, to be co-learners with them. The whole expectation that parents should know what they're doing and should be perfect—that they shouldn't be alcoholics, that they shouldn't have a bad temper, that they shouldn't hurt their children—is both unfortunate and erroneous. The system isn't set up for that. Children are not born into the world to perfect parents who give them everything they need. Instead, it's for you to enter into this world and to understand that all the weaknesses, all the ignorance, and all the pain and suffering were really part of the curriculum for *all* of you to be learning. Sometimes it takes many years to come to this realization.

Your first curriculum is the relationship you contracted with your parents and your family of origin. Your brothers and sisters, your grandparents, your relatives are all a part of the curriculum. This curriculum involves pain, illusion, ignorance, and suffering at the hands of others—as well as causing the suffering and pain of others. This is crucial to understand, because, as you will discover, you have mysteriously re-created those original relationships (with your parents and family) in your marriage, in your work situations, and in your friendships. Like the Buddhists teach, the wheel just keeps going round and round—until someone decides to stop it. *Now it's time for you to end the endless cycle of pain.*

Creating the Parent You Never Had

When you examine your history bank, you see all the hurts, all the damage. You recognize that you were denied the love and support and understanding that you needed. Now you take on the responsibility for becoming the parent you never had. You decide to begin giving yourself what no one else was ever able to give to you. You become responsible for creating and attracting the people in your life who can support you and help you. First, you must get in touch with your sadness and anger, and know whom the resentment and hurt are really directed towards. You need to go into your history bank and understand the events where you were passive and couldn't respond. You need to learn to reframe those events and give yourself new response mechanisms.

Because of your parents' programming and conditioning, try as they might your parents could never have been the parents that you really deserved to have.

Elaine came into a group because she was in a relationship where she felt more alone than as if she had been living by herself. Everything was more important than Elaine was in her current relationship. It took her several months to realize that this problem was related to her childhood. While growing up, Elaine's mother was seldom home and was emotionally unavailable. Her mother's role in the community was more important than being home for dinner. In the evening, rather than preparing dinner she would send Elaine and her brother and sister to a coffee shop down the street. At age ten, Elaine was left to fend for herself, plus she was responsible for her siblings. And, if something went wrong while her mother was gone, she was criticized. When Elaine began examining her history bank, she got in touch with how much she resented having so much responsibility at such an early age. As she began listening to her feelings, she realized how unfair it was of her mother to be gone every night—and equally unfair for her to expect Elaine to do her job. She needed a mother who was present and interested in her life. During group sessions, Elaine practiced many dialogues where she took on the role of the good mother. She would tell Elaine that she cared about her and how important she was to her. She would ask Elaine to share her feelings and reassure her that she was truly interested and would be there to support her. Just the act of being in a women's group and having other women listen to her evoked a whole new experience of how a good mother might respond to a child. Now feeling supported, she began paying attention to her own emotions and chose to be around nurturing women.

You must stand up for the child within you. You're going to become an emotional parent to this emotional child within. You're going to go through re-parenting. Internally, you're taking responsibility to be that parent. That's not going to be enough, however. You also need to create a healing environment in your interpersonal relationships in which you will build an external emotional parent to make up for what you didn't receive from your biological and historical parents.2

Along the way, you will learn about the adult who is connected to the wisdom, the love, and the power to direct this process of healing. You are going to learn to be the parent you wanted and didn't have. You are going to give to this child what it needs. You are going to correct the ignorance of the scripts you inherited from your parents, the erroneous belief systems. You will transcend the conditioning of ignorance that you inherited from your culture and which gave you the false pictures of who and what you are.

Marriage and the Curriculum of Pain

In this stage of the journey, intimate relationships can be painful. There's a lot of fear and anxiety. Most of the time, you are processing your relationship in struggle. If you're lucky, there's *flow,* maybe, 25% of the time. In marriage counseling, it is quite common to find both partners dealing with enlightenment through pain. Each has inherited a curriculum from his or her parents and lifelong-conditioning. The challenge is to bring about the healing of the original historical conditions through healing the marriage. The original pain and hurts have been recreated in the marriage. The couple must become aware of how they re-wound each other. They must choose to stretch and change and to alter how they respond to each other.

It's not unusual to find that one of the pair is not willing to do the necessary work. Many men will not do their work as long as their wives are there, because they will just stay in denial and disassociation, so they're not going to change. Sometimes, the only thing that wakes them up to the process is the threat of their spouse suddenly moving out or asking for a divorce.

De-Roling Your Parents

In enlightenment through pain, you recognize both the strengths and weaknesses of your historical parents, and you choose to create *emotional parents of choice*, men and women—peers or mentors—who can give you nurturing support and validation in ways that were impossible to receive from your parents.

You begin to realize that even though you can't change the way your parents treated you, you can choose to treat yourself differently.

Now you begin to recognize that as a child you suffered from your parents' ignorance. You acknowledge the pain they caused. Often they were not very evolved. They were far from perfect. In fact, they were in need of learning not only how to parent you, but also how to parent themselves – for parents cannot give you what they themselves have not received. Yes, it's true you suffered at their hands. And over time, you will learn to emotionally accept them without blaming them or rejecting yourself. This is part of your healing.

You can forgive your parents, knowing their conditioning, because you can take care of the child within you. You can forgive them because you are no longer dependent on them. Then, you were in the dependency role and reaped the effects of their history. But now you have the chance to take responsibility for your own child and to create a new set of emotional parents. Will you make that choice? Will you forgive them—which means to release the need to blame them—and now take responsibility for *you*? At first, this may seem impossible, when you remember all the pain your child suffered. But it is the first step of your healing and is a fundamental part of the curriculum of enlightenment through pain.

Releasing and Forgiving

Much of the core work of enlightenment through pain is in releasing old negative feelings, forgiving others for the pain they may have caused you, and accepting them exactly as they are.

Releasing

Constantly replaying old negative feelings—anger, rage, hurt, resentment, grief, sadness, frustration or jealousy—will keep you stuck. Releasing means that you are ready to let go of these feelings and not have them be a part of your daily consciousness. This is a crucial step towards healing.

Releasing these negative feelings does not mean that you are necessarily ready to forgive those who caused you pain and suffering, or that you are willing to open your heart to those people. Releasing these feelings also doesn't mean forgetting what happened. Instead, it means accepting responsibility and letting go of the victim status—

being willing to let go of the grip of the negative emotions that have affected you throughout your life.

When you choose to release, you have made a decision that you no longer want to see yourself as a victim, and you are through with blaming others. You now understand what you need for yourself. You know what was missing. You can validate and acknowledge your feelings, and express the pain. This frees you, so you can let the pain go.

Here is the best process for releasing, along with an example—begin by clearly remember the event. Bring the memory up into your consciousness. For example, Carole as a young child had a recurring dream that a fire broke out in her bedroom as she was sleeping. She would awake terrified, not knowing what to do, and would climb out of the window onto the fire escape. It's important to become aware of all the feelings, beliefs and judgments that come up for you around that memory. Although Carole was in a panic, she told herself not to call out to her parents, fearing that they would be angry for waking them in the middle of the night.

Next, recall the things that were told to you in connection with this event, as well as the things you may have told yourself. Carole was never told not to wake her parents; however, she was convinced that they would be angry if she were to awaken them. The enlightenment through pain then comes through re-framing. You look at what you really needed in this situation, what you would like to have been told – as compared to what actually happened and what you heard in reality. Ask yourself, How would I have wanted to experience this differently? Carole would have wanted to awake from her nightmare and be able to call out to her parents for help and be comforted and reassured.

Once you have brought all this into awareness and know what you want to release, you now have choices to make (a matter of will): Are you willing to take responsibility for your experience—even your pain? Are you willing to give yourself what you needed then, or do you want to have someone else give this to you? Are you willing to receive it from somebody else? Will you now release those old feelings and beliefs? How long do you want to hold on to them? Are you ready to let them go now?

Imagine that your mental and emotional house is like a refrigerator, full of soggy vegetables, rancid meat and sour milk that have been sitting on the shelves for years. On the kitchen counter, there are bags of fresh produce—vegetables, eggs and milk—that are only part of what is available from the wonderful markets in the world. But until you empty your refrigerator, you have no space to put the fresh produce. There is a great table waiting to be set, and there are people waiting to share the feast. You cannot create the delicious meal you want or invite the people with whom you'd love to share it—if those bags of fresh food sit on the counter long enough, they too will go bad.

You have held on to certain painful memories so that one day you could become aware of your real needs that have gone unmet—and be able to choose to meet those needs yourself.

The point is that *release is not loss.* It is simply a process of letting go of the negative thoughts and beliefs that have prevented you from accessing your good. Part of enlightenment through pain is emptying out your refrigerator of stored pain.

Forgiving

After learning to release the old negative feelings, it will eventually become time to learn to forgive. In forgiveness, you take responsibility for being the architect of your life and your scripts. You reach the point where you can say the following:

All that has offended me, I forgive. I am ready to bring the memories up, work through the feelings, get in touch with what was withheld from me, and give it to myself. I'm ready to forgive and release those people who abused me or couldn't give me what I needed, because now I can take care of and protect myself.

Please understand that forgiving doesn't mean saying that something you know was wrong is now right. It's not agreement with what happened. Forgiving, like releasing, means that you have identified your needs and that you take responsibility for caring for yourself.

For instance, in the past you may have experienced that no one listened to you, and you may still be angry and resentful about not being heard. Your feelings may have been minimized, or when you shared them you were interrupted or simply ignored and disregarded. Experiencing your anger in the present gives you information about what you wanted and didn't receive, or what you got and didn't want. It tells you what you need to pay attention to and how to take care of yourself and get your needs met now. As you begin to identify your needs, you will begin to choose to be with people who listen to you and support you.

In a way, forgiveness is a very "selfish" process. By releasing your negative emotions and forgiving others, you feel more positive about yourself and can accept more good into your life.

Ultimately, you are able to forgive because you can identify your needs and respond to them yourself. You can give to yourself what your parents couldn't give you, and you are now capable of receiving it from others. In this way, you no longer have to remember the painful past.

Another group member, Marilee, remembered that when she was a little girl and disagreed with her mother, her mother would abruptly stop talking to her—just cut her off. The only way Marilee could reconnect with her mother was to "admit" she was wrong and that her mother was right. It was only then that her mother would "forgive" her. That's not forgiveness. Forgiveness doesn't mean saying something was right when you believe it was wrong, or saying somebody didn't hurt you when you know they did. Forgiveness is an honest acknowledgment of *what is*. Because you don't want to stay in the victim role and you don't want to continue feeling separate and alone, you let go of the negative emotions that are destructive for your physical and emotional well being.

When you choose to let go of the resentments and hurts from the past, you can feel better about yourself and more connected to others. In order to get out of the cycle of pain and hurt, you need to let go and forgive. In so doing, you are taking responsibility for your past so that you can create a new present. You cannot have a new experience in the present if you are attached to the past with anger, resentment and hurt.

In forgiveness, you develop the ability to accept your parents just as they were and stop emotionally resisting who they were and how they treated you. You stop fighting the unfairness. This is not to say that what they did was right, but more positively, it's to acknowledge them *as learners*. You may have had the expectation that yours would be perfect parents, that they knew what to do and you were to be in the receiving role and follow them. But in enlightenment through pain, you realize that this was not the script to be lived. The *real* script was that *they were learners with you*. You discover that the parent/child relationship is a joint learning process.

The idea of perfect parents is an unhelpful expectation. Learning how to parent rightly *is* an appropriate aspiration. Your parents were not supposed to automatically know how to be parents.

If you have ignorant parents operating with a limited understanding of what parenting is about, how can you expect evolved, emotional responses from them? It's impossible. Forgiveness means that you realize that *you were all there to learn from each other.* Is that painful learning? Yes, it's enlightenment through pain. Learning is what it's all about.

Letting Go of Judgments and Resentments

Enlightenment through pain is also the stage where you let go of judgments. You learn discrimination and come to understand what you're responsible for. You learn to let go of taking responsibility for other people or wanting to manipulate them in order to meet certain needs.

Judgments are self-fulfilling prophecies that keep you separate from yourself and others.

You begin to understand that on a fundamental level, your parents' *intentions* towards you were good, but their programming, social conditioning and belief systems did not support them in carrying out those intentions. As you acknowledge that you cannot always do or support what is your own ideal for yourself, and begin to realize how much you are affected and controlled by your own programming and beliefs, you can begin to release the need to judge. Instead, you can take the attitude—*I accept my mistakes. I accept my parents' mistakes. We are learners, not masters.*

As you begin to accept yourself as a learner who can make mistakes and accept the fact that you need *self-correction*—just as your parents did—you can then choose to take responsibility for your choices and become proactive, rather than being reactive and judgmental. Here, you let go of judging yourself and others. You understand that when you accept yourself, you are in a process of growth and change.

In humility, you understand that it was your programming that caused your suffering and that it was your parents' programming that caused their suffering. You realize that each and every person is responsible for himself or herself, in a process of awakening and becoming conscious. You learn to release and let go of old hurts and resentments. You understand that like attracts like, and you are ready to release the pain in your life. Humility is an important attitude for you to hold in enlightenment through pain. But humility is not self-abnegation. Instead, it is born out of the recognition that your scripts have long controlled your attitudes and your thinking.

You have to go through a sufficient amount of pain and awareness before you have the will to love yourself—before you can discover the will inside of you. Self-love is not a feeling—it is a choice.

As you see other people—like your parents—stuck in their scripts, any arrogance or self-righteousness you may have once held turns to humility and compassion. Now you understand how long and how much effort you have expended and can appreciate how much work and time it will take for others or your parents to heal and change. Humility comes from recognizing all you have had to learn and unlearn in order to move forward in your life.

Staying on Course

You have come far enough in your experience now that you have some compassion for your own suffering. You have done a measure of forgiveness, both of yourself and those who have caused you suffering. You've realized that you are a being with physical, emotional and mental needs, with a personal history. A great deal of self-correction has occurred. You've chosen to re-frame your past and to re-parent yourself. You have committed to the process of healing, found a guide, and embarked on the journey of your soul. You know that the journey will not be easy, but you're determined to see it through.

Things may get worse before they get better.

Besides making sure you get the personal therapeutic support that you need and deserve as you go through enlightenment through pain, there are many other things you can do for yourself. Many valuable books are now available that can help you stay on course. Take the time to feed your soul during this time. Make yourself your first priority.

Here are some guidelines that will help you stay the course, to keep you moving forward on your soul's journey during the time of enlightenment through pain.

"The Window"

Picture an image of the Sun—which is light, love, beauty, harmony, joy and wisdom. (Some people even call this God.) You, on the other hand, are like a window. Your purpose is to let this light, love, and beauty of the Sun shine and be expressed through you. But because of all the suffering and pain you have endured, your window has bars or blinds that block out some of the light. If your pain has been especially traumatic, you may even have drapes on your window. Because of the ignorance and illusion covering the window, very little of the light and love can come through you. Enlightenment through pain is about taking the bars off your window, taking down the drapes, so that the essential nature of who you are can radiate and shine through.

The Importance of a Support Group

You don't endure enlightenment through pain alone. You can face the pain with support, with a viewpoint larger than your own. This makes healing possible. Part of your work is to connect yourself with other people who are going through the healing process themselves. This does not necessarily have to be "group therapy," but you will want to find a support group that is attuned to the special needs of enlightenment through pain.

Community is a basic human need. You will need a "community" or group of people who are equally committed to their own and each other's healing and growth. In this community, you will develop the vital skill of speaking and listening deeply to each other. You will be heard. And you will hear and receive others at a soul level.

Affirmations for Stage One

Throughout your journey, affirmations can be extremely helpful in keeping you on course. The reason to use affirmations in enlightenment through pain is that you will have been programmed by old painful thoughts, and you need to constantly give yourself new thoughts to replace them. Your mind will continue to operate on automatic until you tell it to stop.

Affirmations are positive statements that assert a desire to be a certain way. Affirmations are always in the present, always positive and always stated as if they are already operating in your life. Their purpose is to replace the negative programming with positive thoughts that support positive outcomes on physical, emotional and mental levels in our life. The basic principle is that to change the outside you must first change the inside. Thought creates outcome.

An affirmation is like a seed, a new thought that you put into the earth of your mind. Through affirming it out loud, repeatedly, you nurture that new thought until it becomes a shoot and eventually a flower in your garden. Releasing and forgiving will pull out the weeds.

An affirmation is a positive thought that you affirm in the present so you can make it true for your life.

It is best to say your affirmations out loud. The spoken word has the power to change your field of energy as you speak. In saying the words of an affirmation, you are literally creating the reality you want. For instance, in using a releasing affirmation, your thoughts and feelings are energetically releasing the old thought-forms as you speak. This also energizes and empowers you in the process. Through repetition, you are planting the new thought in your conscious and unconscious mind and giving it energy until it takes root and ultimately manifests what you want in your life.

Below are powerful affirmations you can use for your journey during enlightenment through pain. While you are working on your own re-programming, I would recommend saying many of these daily, a loud. This will support the analytical and emotional part of the re-programming process. I also strongly recommend that you *memorize* one or two of these affirmations each week. This way, when you hit one of those moments when you become reactive or negative, you will have a more positive thought to think and say aloud. This will help shift you into a higher level of awareness and being in that moment.

- I am a learner.
- I am capable of change.
- I accept my mistakes.
- I am in a process of healing and change.
- I mentally accept the possibility that I can learn from this experience of pain.
- I mentally accept the possibility that I could heal from this experience of hurt and suffering.
- I know that release is magnetic.[4] Through the act of release, I now draw to myself my own. I now fully and freely release. I loose and let go. I let go and grow. I let go and trust.
- All that has offended me I forgive. I am ready to bring the memories up, work through the feelings, get in touch with what was withheld and give it to myself.
- I'm ready to forgive and release those people who couldn't give me what I needed or who abused me, because now I can take care of myself.
- I accept responsibility for my life.
- I release the need to judge, criticize and contend. Instead, I choose to praise, support and validate.
- I accept responsibility for the re-programming of my parents' scripts.
- I release the need to blame.
- I accept responsibility for being the parent I have always desired.

- In accepting my parents and myself, I am enlightened and healed.

- I emotionally accept myself with all my scripts, all my

- programming, all my beliefs, all my mistakes, all my weaknesses and strengths, all my failures and successes. I make the commitment to accept the whole package, from the consciousness of a learner.
- I am here for the journey. I am here to grow.
- I am responsive to the child within me. (Love Notes)
- I take the good from each relationship. I let the rest go. (Catherine Ponder)

The Road Ahead

Enlightenment through pain is not forever. And yet, it is a place that you are likely to revisit at various moments of your life. Make no mistake, enlightenment through pain demands that you work through all the curriculum of your past. To move successfully through all seven stages of your life's journey, you need to be very thorough about completing your work in enlightenment through pain. There are no shortcuts here. But don't worry. If you have not resolved something from your past, something of which you may not even be conscious, it will eventually surface and give you the opportunity to resolve the issue that is still causing you pain.

Don't be in a hurry to accelerate your process. Through opening your awareness to pain, the consequences could cause a divorce, a change of career, or re-evaluation of your relationships with your family.

You might wonder how long it takes to complete Stage One and be able to move to Stage Two. There is no way to predict the amount of time you need, as this is an individual matter. It will depend on how deeply you want to delve into your history, how wounded you are and how much time and energy you want to devote to your healing. Working this process is a matter of gaining new insights and being able to make behavioral changes. You may discover you need many hours of nurturing and support to re-examine your past and gain the understanding and the validation you didn't receive as a child. There may even be times in Stage One when everything gets worse before it can get better.

Through opening your awareness to pain, the consequences could cause a divorce, a change of career, or a re-evaluation of your relationships with your family. Just because you are going through this process doesn't necessarily mean that those around will understand. They may think or feel that you are acting quite differently. They may even feel threatened, defensive or downright hostile. The fallout of this process can cause a ripple effect creating more challenges than you initially envisioned, demanding an extraordinary expenditure of time and energy. If you have made the decision to heal, your patience and persistence—along with your hard work—will keep you moving on your journey. It takes courage and it takes help.

Self-love begins when you have made the commitment to process for change and growth and healing.

It isn't unusual for someone to be in Stage One for one to three years. This would not be considered a very long time to be actively working on enlightenment through pain. It's important to remember there is no need to accelerate the process beyond what you are capable of achieving. You are worth the time, commitment and effort. It is all part of your spiritual journey.

Don't be surprised or alarmed if you find that you fall back into Stage One when you enter other stages of the journey. When you work on other areas of your life, Stage One has a way of resurfacing. Know you are on a journey that has many pauses. You now understand that a momentary return to Stage One need not overwhelm you.

The road ahead is taking you from the pain of the past into the open moment of the present. When you enter Stage Two you will expand on all the insights and wisdom you gained in Stage One. You will be grateful that you recognized the opportunity—and spent the time—to create a strong foundation by re-parenting and responding to your inner child as well as practicing the process of re-framing, releasing and forgiveness. Now you will feel prepared to build a positive new self-concept.

Questions to Contemplate

In *enlightenment through pain*, as you look back over your life, you will be re-evaluating and re-thinking everything. Nothing can be taken for granted. Ask yourself these questions:

- What parts of my history do I still need to release?
- Where am I holding on to negative feelings from the past?
- Who do I still need to forgive?
- Have I fully committed to my own healing?
- Do I have the support I need for this stage of my life?

End Notes

[1] Acknowledgement and thanks to Wayne Dyer for the phrase 'enlightenment through pain'. He used it in an early '90s lecture, and it just clicked. I have used it ever since.

[2] Historically, parents or "family of origin" are not necessarily biological parents. They are the ones who were actually your primary caregivers in your early years.

[3] From *Love Notes* by Joyce Strum.

[4] From *The Dynamic Laws Of Prosperity* by Catherine Ponder.

Stage 2

Developing a Positive Self-Concept

I'm here to do the journey.

In this stage, we cover Choosing to Love Yourself, Letting Go of the "Be Perfect" Script, Learning to Say and Hear "No", and Self-Validation.

The View From Here

Stage Two feels like a breath of fresh air in comparison to the toxic fumes of negativity in Stage One. The fog of depression dissipates. The clouds of sadness lift and the whole atmosphere changes. It isn't necessary to blame or seek sympathy as a poor helpless victim. You're on the path of healing and change.

Here, you care enough about yourself to know you are worthy, and that your life is worth examining and understanding. You have placed a value on suffering as an important part of your journey of awakening. You no longer run from pain; you embrace it and choose to understand its meaning and importance for your life and growth. Pain has become your spiritual teacher.

I'm here to grow. I've made a statement about my life and its values; I am important. I have value.

During Stage One, no matter how much you desired or thought you deserved love and support, you seemed to attract pain and sorrow. In the past, you were more interested and in need of sympathy and support—which meant you were incapable of forgetting your pain. It is only when you have worked your pain sufficiently that you're ready to begin building a positive self-concept. This doesn't mean you won't find yourself back in enlightenment through pain reviewing your history bank occasionally—this can happen at any time during the journey.

In Stage Two you are no longer overwhelmed by other people's pain because you have confronted and worked through your own pain. You've gone through the dark expanses of your memory bank and come out on the other end—into the light. You have traveled through hurt and disappointment. You can understand the fear of those entering the darkness for the first time. You're less judgmental and feel compassion for those around you—for your own struggle as well as theirs.

You feel compassion for your own struggle and for those around you.

By this point in the journey you have created a large enough emotional vacuum to have the capacity and the strength of will to build a positive self-concept. This is when you choose to accept all your strengths and weaknesses. Now that your will is positioned to allow you to love yourself unconditionally—the process of healing brings the realization that it isn't necessary to be bound to scripts and messages from the past. You have the desire to choose and write a powerful script that builds your self-confidence and positive self-regard. Letting go of self-defeating thoughts leads to a more positive and empowering mindset.

It is therefore important to create a supportive environment that teaches you to discriminate between your old self-concept and your new emerging positive self. Here, you find that when you respect yourself you attract people who respect and validate you. You surround yourself with people who love and care about you. As your self-esteem increases, you release the need to judge and criticize others. You accept them, like yourself, as learners who are here to grow through painful experiences.

The Transition from Stage One to Stage Two

The transition from Stage One to Stage Two is only possible after a sufficient amount of work has been done in enlightenment through pain. In Stage One, the predominant feeling was of self-righteous indignation that generated the self-talk of fault-finding and resentment. You learned that pain brought you face-to-face with an enormous task—the task of expanding your awareness and creating a larger and more positive container of self so that you could heal the past and its effects on the present.

To accomplish this transition, four important transformations had to occur in Stage One. First, you moved from numbness and denial to giving yourself permission to feel the pain and hurt. Second, you chose to focus on the past and remembered your suffering and unhappiness. You allowed yourself to communicate your history with all its disappointments, failures and frustrations. In doing this, your feelings were heard, supported and validated. Third, you gave yourself the parent you always wanted and didn't have—you became the emotional parent of choice. And finally, you began the process of forgiving and releasing the past.

When Margaret came into her group she was firmly entrenched in Stage One. It took her more than two years to work enlightenment through pain to the point where she was able to move into Stage Two.

Margaret always felt that her mother wore a mask of pretense and indifference and didn't care about her. Only positive feelings were to be expressed and accepted. She received the message from her mother that it was necessary to suppress all negative feelings. During Margaret's Stage One re-parenting, she gave herself a mother who cared about all her internal feelings—a mother who really wanted to know and hear her pain as well as her joy. She also worked through being supercritical of her husband and blaming him for everything that went wrong in their marriage. Margaret made a major shift when she decided to be emotionally honest with him about a covert affair. And, most importantly, things really began changing when she decided to take full responsibility for her feelings of unhappiness and insecurity. When she forgave herself for her deceit and released the unreasonable expectations of her husband, Margaret was able to rewrite her self-concept.

Tim's entrance into Stage One happened when his two stepchildren left home and he made the sudden decision to leave his marriage of 15 years. He felt that he was nothing more than a financial provider and that his family had been frivolous with his money. During enlightenment through pain he discovered why he had been living all those years in a loveless marriage. It took him a long time to get past the memories of his own stepmother who had beaten and locked him in a closet. After Tim addressed his denial about his anger, he took responsibility for not telling his wife about his deeply buried resentment and stopped blaming her for not understanding his needs. After developing the good parent in Stage One, he learned to reassure himself that it was safe to express his feelings. Now, entering Stage Two, he was ready to build a new self-concept.

Now you can take responsibility for healing your pain.

Perhaps you have also seen yourself as one of those people to whom misfortune occurs; one of those people who always come up short—where your life feels unfair, unjust and unhappy. In Stage Two, it's important to have released those negative attitudes and emotions. You can no longer feel yourself at the mercy of circumstances. Instead, you have the energy and strong desire to affirm and see your life in a positive way. You have learned enough about your past scripts to identify those that support you from those you need to release and change. You are in the privileged position to choose new scripts that can help you create and expand your self-concept and self-esteem.

Stage Two Work

Choosing to Love Yourself

Once you release the negativity of the past you have more energy available to live in the present. You make new choices. Your will is positioned for loving yourself unconditionally. You accept your strengths, weaknesses, successes and failures. This is the foundation from which all change and growth occurs. Unconditional love is an attitude, a choice, and a decision. The affect is a warm, nurturing, caring, and compassionate feeling.

Self-love is a choice of will and is not selfish.

The "will" acts first, then the feeling follows.

No part of me is too imperfect to reject. Now I really love myself. I'm building a concept of myself as acceptable, with my pluses and minuses. I'm actually beginning to enjoy being with myself. Each morning I greet myself with the sense that I love myself, I'm happy to be alive.

I'm beginning to replace judgments and criticisms with validating affirmations. I'm worthy of love and respect. I surround myself with people who love and care about me. The child in me is absolutely thrilled with all this positive validation.

Understanding the Three Levels of Unconditional Love

There are three levels of unconditional love—physical, emotional and mental. The physical level is when you choose to love and accept your body, to see its beauty and wisdom. You can look into the mirror and see a magnificent human being. You let go of the social and media stereotypes and recognize that this body is for your healing growth and enlightenment on this physical plane.

Many women acquire a poor self-concept in childhood. For example, Nikki heard her mother go through the same ritual every morning. When her mother was dressing she would look at herself in the mirror and say, "I am ugly." She would point to her nose and say that it was too long and that her hair was limp and dull. Or, that her hips were too broad and her breasts too small. There was always something which made her less than or imperfect. The imperfections she perceived were totally a fabrication of her mind. In fact, her friends and family told her how beautiful she was and what a gorgeous body she had. Nikki's mother didn't hear those comments and surely didn't feel it internally. So her perception of herself was that she was ugly—not pretty enough and not good enough. One day, Nikki recognized she had followed in her mother's footsteps. As she was dressing and looking into the mirror,

Accept yourself unconditionally without reservation.

her daughter Anne began mimicking her and said, "Oh I'm so ugly, I can't bear to look at myself in the mirror." Nikki was startled into the realization that she was passing on to her daughter her mother's script. She understood how painful it was to be that self-critical. Based on this awareness, Nikki made a commitment to accept and love her body so that her daughter Anne wouldn't inherit the painful script she had.

This is not only true for women—it can be true for men, as well. Tom was a big, handsome, burly guy who was terribly self-conscious about his physical appearance. After much agonizing, he decided he would feel better if he could get rid of the fat around his mid-section and thighs. As a quick fix to his lack of self-esteem and poor body concept, he decided to have liposuction. After a painful and uncomfortable surgery, he found it made little difference in his feelings about himself and within a few months he regained most of the weight. When Tom realized that having the surgery didn't solve his problem, he entered a men's group. There he was able to identify the impact on his self-esteem of his father abandoning him as a young boy. He also became aware of his need for a positive fatherly relationship. By experiencing the emotional support and positive feedback from the other men in the group, Tom was able to change his feelings about his body and increase his self-esteem.

It is here that you turn the emotional acceptance up a notch by choosing to actively nurture a positive self-regard.

On the emotional level, you choose to nurture and care for yourself, to have an appreciation and positive self-regard; you experience feelings of warmth and tenderness, patience and reassurance. Ella was working hard to support herself and her autistic daughter. She sought help when she found it was almost impossible to bear the guilt of having a difficult child. To make matters worse, her husband blamed her for this untenable position and was extremely critical of her. Before Ella was able to move into Stage Two, she had to acknowledge her feelings of grief and disappointment at having a mentally challenging child. She had to express her anger toward her husband for his lack of emotional support. And, more importantly, she had to forgive herself. Now she was ready to give and receive the unconditional love on the emotional level she needed to build her positive self-regard.

On a mental level, you choose to praise and support—to release the need to judge, criticize and find fault. You develop tolerance and understanding. You focus on what's right and not what's wrong. George was a successful businessman despite his lack of a college education. Regardless of how well the business did, there was always self-doubt and criticism of how little he knew—he assumed that he had been lucky. Never did he feel it was his business acumen that made his business successful. When he entered Stage Two, he let go of his faultfinding. He replaced each negative judgment with words of praise. He eventually affirmed that education doesn't necessarily make a person smart and that his level of intelligence was equal to, if not better than, most college graduates.

Broadening Your Consciousness

In Stage Two, both men and women—in slightly different ways—have to separate doing and being, especially as each relates to self-worth.

Before I do anything or try to achieve anything, I know that I am lovable, whole and acceptable. Because I am here, because I breathe, I am enough. I am valuable.

Self-acceptance means having a central core that doesn't depend on other people's judgments or opinions. The result is true self-confidence. Unconditional acceptance provides the strength to maintain a sense of security, despite opposition or disapproval. Jane wanted to go back to school and finish her degree. Her husband was totally against the idea. In fact, he judged her by saying that she was a bad mother and was abandoning her children. Since he was a good provider, he couldn't understand why she wanted to return to school. Jane was so overwhelmed by her husband's disapproval that she backed down. Over the next few months, Jane gained ten pounds, which forced her to seek help—so she joined a group. It was there that she realized the weight gain was the result of her not going back to school and that she had substituted eating for meeting her needs for growth.

Finally she decided to enroll in spite of her husband's judgments and, within a month, the weight was gone. She finally communicated that if he wanted to be with her, and keep their family together, it was necessary for him to accept her decision to return to school.

People with positive self-esteem can receive feedback, evaluate it, and discern between what is valid and worthy of consideration, rather than fold when someone doesn't support or agree with them. The capability of being unguarded allows for the acceptance of new input that can then be incorporated into one's self. At the same time, it enables one to say "no" to suggestions and ideas that don't fit. There is no sense of being afraid of losing outer approval or of hurting someone's feelings.

It takes a very strong ego to accept feedback as information, not as criticism or rejection, and to accept feedback without getting defensive or rationalizing it away. When Jack came into a group he was a person who had to have everything his way and who had a very hard time receiving feedback from his wife

You don't see yourself as superior and others inferior or less than.

and children. As he began to dismantle some of his defenses, and learned to love and accept himself whether he was right or wrong, he became more open to receiving alternate points of view.

Your consciousness expands and broadens when you let go of self-righteousness and arrogance. You are not out to be right or prove others wrong. You accept differences and appreciate the uniqueness of every individual at each point in their journey.

The Internal Voice of the Good Mother and Good Father

Developing self-esteem in Stage Two is choosing to replace the negative scripts you inherited from your parents and parental figures with newer, emotionally supported voices. These new mental discourses are the voices of the "good mother" and "good father," which become your emotional parents. These internal voices assure you of a commitment to always be present. They communicate total respect for who you are, despite your failures and weaknesses. These voices further remind you that you are intelligent, loving and strong.

The script of the "good mother" voice replaces the fear of abandonment and fear of being judged. The "good mother" voice reassures unconditional love and acceptance. It is especially important that women release the negative messages which foster self-doubt and hatred directed inward. Remember Nikki, who had to replace the negative script she learned from her mother regarding ugliness and competitiveness with a new script that she was unique and beautiful. Women who choose to create an internal maternal voice of unconditional love—one that is trustworthy and present in joy as well as sadness—develop a secure foundation for positive self-esteem.

The voice of the "good father" is one of respect and positive regard. The "good father" does not communicate put-downs or comparisons. He doesn't judge. He doesn't destroy respect after a defeat. Jake felt less than his brother because of a competition that his father had set up when he was a boy. He was resentful when his father would compliment his brother and would repeatedly tell Jake he wasn't measuring up. In Stage Two, he developed an internal good father who showed him respect, who told him he didn't need to be in competition with anyone and that he was good enough by himself.

Individual situations require some expansion of this general pattern. These are the issues that drag down self-esteem and self-concept.

Women might tend to be more afraid of abandonment and being left alone while men suffer most from fear of failure, letting people down, and not measuring up. The voice of the "good father" validates through wins and losses. It encourages persisting and offers words of comfort that provide the strength to face failure. It replaces the voice of threat, intimidation, ridicule, or shame that allows the building of self-esteem. Men also fear abandonment and therefore need the self-talk to support them in that regard, while women—especially those in high pressure, high performance careers—need to deal with the fear of failure.

Self-Talk

In Stage Two, you constantly talk to yourself in new ways. You become self-supportive. You encourage yourself. You believe in yourself. You tell yourself that you deserve to be happy. You believe you deserve good things.

As passionately as you relived your pains and hurts during Stage One, now you affirm how much you love yourself. The result is that you really glow. There is a new light that shines through your eyes. When you become aware of your self-talk and recognize that you can choose the way it sounds, you want to make it as positive as possible.

Negative Self-Talk:

How could I do that? I can't believe the way I messed up! What are people going to think? Oh, my God, I looked so stupid. I've never been so embarrassed. I want to crawl in a hole and never come out. I will never walk into that place again. What did I expect? What a loser!

Positive Self-Talk:

Wow, that was a new experience, a real first. I was nervous, but I was courageous. I sure got a lot of feedback and, boy, is that going to help me the next time. I am really proud of myself because I had the courage to step out there and do something for the first time. I got great compliments. I could see that people wanted me to succeed. They understood it was my first time. I learned so much.

It's important to note that positive self-talk does not mean being a Pollyanna. The difference is in the way the events are framed. For example:

Negative Self-Talk:

Getting married and divorced four times means I'm a loser. I don't think there are any good men out there. I feel like an old hag since I'm going through my change. How can I expect anything more from relationships?

Positive Self-Talk:

Every relationship I've been in has been a major stepping stone in my life. I learned so much from each one. I grew as a person. I love men, and I love being in a relationship. My partners helped me work through stuff from my childhood. I treasure everyone I've loved. Relationships are like mirrors reflecting my soul's growth.

Once you have the guidelines that can help you think and reframe things more appropriately, you have the capacity to take control of your self-talk.

Letting Go of the "Be Perfect" Script

With a new, emerging self-concept, you might want to know: "What are my new rights? Have I given myself the freedom to choose the 'scripts' that support a more expansive and positive self? "First you will want to let go of the "be perfect" script which usually reads like this: I can't do anything unless I do it perfectly. Since I would probably make a mistake the first time I tried something new, why take a chance and attempt anything unfamiliar?

While growing up, Rhonda demonstrated a talent for art and dreamt that she would be an artist one day. After graduating from high school, she decided not to apply to a fine arts program because of her fear of rejection and failure, although it was her dream to be an artist. Rather, she chose to become a nail technician. Learning to do nails was easy for Rhonda, although within a few years of working she became restless and bored. What she secretly desired was to pursue her artistic nature. What troubled Rhonda was that to actualize her dream would take years and there was no guarantee that she would be successful. While in a group process, Rhonda became aware that she had to rewrite her "be perfect" script before she could realize her dream.

Several interrelated fears operate here: fear of failure, fear of making a mistake, fear of losing face, and fear of not getting approval. These factors keep you stuck in what you already know and prevent you from trying things that are unknown.

Bill's story differs by demonstrating his inability to ask for guidance, which had, in the process, put his wife and himself in danger. They went sailing with some friends who were experienced sailors and had a wonderful time. After this excursion, Bill decided he wanted to take his wife sailing by himself. Since Bill had no experience or understanding of how to sail, and hadn't felt it necessary to ask for training or assistance, the boat capsized and he and his wife nearly drowned. In fact, it wasn't until he remembered this incident that he acknowledged how difficult it was for him to ask for assistance and direction.

A similar script might read: I can't ask for help because doing so would reveal that I'm not already perfect. I can't admit that I don't know the answer. It's a sign of weakness to ask for assistance, direction or guidance.

If you are afraid of being revealed as weak or less than perfect, you may feel it necessary to develop multiple facades. Exposing any self-perceived weakness or limitation might be embarrassing. However, maintaining these masks usually causes greater entrapment and generally leads to poor judgment calls.

Letting go of the "be perfect" script releases a heavy burden—the feeling that you're obligated to do things perfectly the first time. You acknowledge and accept that you are a learner in the process of self-correction. You know you need help. In fact, you realize it is a sign of strength and wisdom to reach out and ask for assistance or support when doing something new.

For a long time, Chris could not admit that she was in an unhappy marriage. It was very important for her to maintain the image of perfection to the outer world—it was better to be unhappy than admit a mistake. When she got to the breaking point, she finally sought counseling. This was an enormous hurdle for her to overcome because she had to admit she needed help. Once Chris became familiar with the process, she realized it wasn't a sign of weakness to seek help but a sign of strength. After some time, she felt safe to write a new script saying that there will be times when it is perfect to acknowledge what isn't working. Some months later she had the courage to invite her husband to join her for joint counseling sessions where, to her amazement, he was open and willing to address their issues and make the changes to improve their marriage.

Feedback delivered in a respectful manner and by a caring spirit can be difficult to hear as long as the "be perfect" script remains. As with Chris, both she and her husband needed to learn better ways of listening and communicating their needs to one another. Amazingly, neither one of them had learned how to do this while growing up in their families. Now, in their relationship, they had the opportunity to dismantle the "be perfect" script and be honest with each other.

It takes considerable strength and a positive self-esteem to accept constructive criticism.

Taking risks and being less afraid allows you to let go of the fear that others will judge you to be lacking. As you let go of the "know it all" attitude, you gain compassion and patience for yourself and others. Instead of being confined within a box of your own expectations, you open to a greater freedom. The willingness to expose yourself to the possibility of failure by taking risks comes with an increasing ability to accept yourself.

I accept myself as a whole package. I know that I come with weaknesses, strengths, and areas of ignorance and wisdom. I choose to give myself permission to try something new and not succeed. I choose to give myself room to grow.

Accepting Your Feelings

Letting go of stereotypes like "good girls don't get angry" and "big boys don't cry" allows you to accept feelings you ordinarily would have rejected. It is necessary to accept the entire spectrum of your emotions—particularly if you have labeled some feelings either good or bad. When feelings are viewed as sources of information, inappropriate stereotypes and expectations can be released.

Emotions are nothing more than information about what you like and dislike.

Consequently, a man who cries isn't showing weakness, he is indicating that he feels hurt, grieving or showing a symptom of disappointment. This show of feelings contains signals that the man should take care of himself, perhaps by reaching out for support and love or by identifying an old past script that needs to be processed, released or forgiven.

Lee was a 42-year-old man who thought that strong men didn't cry. One day during a session he recalled that his parents hadn't thought enough of him to come to his law school graduation. At the time, he had told himself it really wasn't that important and that it didn't matter, although the group did notice that Lee never showed any emotion on his face and most often spoke in a monotone. Once he realized that this was a defense mechanism covering his feelings of hurt, he broke down and cried. In that moment, Lee exposed all his hurt, anger, disappointment and sadness—which destroyed that old script. When Lee acknowledged his feelings, he affirmed his self-worth and gave himself permission to express all that was inside of him.

You learn not to expect to feel happy all the time.

In Stage Two, you know you are worthy and that all feelings are acceptable as part of the whole. You can look at them as a way of expressing your needs and connecting with others. You develop the flexibility to have a variety of feelings, accepting all of them. Imagine your feelings as compared to the atmospheric conditions at the seashore. One minute the sun comes out and you feel warm and wonderful. Then a cloud covers the sun and you put a shirt on over your swimsuit because you feel chilled. Next, a few drops of rainfall and you wonder whether to stay or pack up and go home. And finally, to your amazement and surprise, the sun bursts forth again and you start thinking about going for a dip in the ocean. By not rejecting your ever-changing feelings, you increase your self-

Feelings are in a constant state of flux.

esteem and self-love and have the confidence to communicate and share who you are.

Getting Your Needs Met

As your self-esteem increases, you develop a broader acceptance of the whole range of your needs and feel more comfortable communicating them. Some of you might have grown up with the expectation that others could read your mind. In fact, some of you went so far as to believe that if someone really loved and cared about you they would instinctively know what your needs were. If they didn't, perhaps you felt that this meant they didn't care or love you. Unfortunately, this becomes a misguided, artificial measure of love against which others invariably fail to measure up.

Alex had been working for a very progressive company. When he was hired, they told him that the quality of life of their employees was paramount. Alex discovered that meant working 80 hours a week—which he did for one year. During that entire year he waited—expecting that they would reward him for his above and beyond behavior. As time passed and nothing was forthcoming from management, he felt unhappy and unappreciated. Rather than tell his superiors how he felt, he started to look for another job. Alex did finally come to his senses and tell his boss what he needed. Upon asking to have his needs met, he got a huge raise and an assistant to help with the workload.

Sylvia, on the other hand, had been married for 15 years and still hadn't received a birthday present from her husband. Each year she would wait and hope that he would come home with something outrageously expensive for her. Her expectation was that if he really loved her he would make the effort. One day Sylvia finally worked up the courage to tell him how important she felt it was

If you ask, most likely the answer will be yes.

for him to buy her a birthday present. He was surprised and felt quite guilty at not meeting her expectation. What she learned from him was that, in his family, birthdays were incidental. From that day forward, Sylvia reminded her husband that her birthday was coming and even gave him a few hints as to what she might like.

With the changes brought about in Stage Two comes the realization that others will not know what you want intuitively. Instead of silently assuming you aren't lovable because someone isn't reading your mind and satisfying your desires, the act of asking provides at least a 50-50 chance of getting your needs met. Now, with your ability to communicate, you get your needs met in a timely and appropriate manner, one that validates your right to be happy and fulfilled.

Learning to Say and Hear "No"

Another right you have as you change your self-concept is your right to say no and feel good about yourself. Chances are that you were taught that saying no meant that you were uncaring. In the past when you said no, you may have seen negative consequences, hurt someone's feelings or experienced someone becoming so angry that they punished you by withholding their love or leaving the relationship.

Sue struggled for many years with this problem by going along with her husband and his family's expectation that they spend every Christmas together. Since she had no family, it seemed unreasonable and uncaring not to want to be with his family, therefore she voiced no objections. What she really wanted was to spend one year with his family and the next year go on a ski vacation or plan something with other friends. Sue was afraid to hurt her husband's family's feelings and was equally fearful of her husband's reaction—worrying that he would either be angry or choose his family over her wishes. She wanted to say no and feel good about herself and still be seen as caring by her husband. Much to her surprise, when she told her husband what she wanted he acknowledged that he too wanted to experience the holidays differently.

It is also difficult—at times almost impossible—to tolerate or hear the word "no." For some, hearing no is synonymous with rejection. Perhaps you associate the word with being unlovable, unwanted, or undesirable. Here in Stage Two you learn that hearing no needn't become a trigger for survival reflexes. Instead, this is the time to be open to receiving information and not feeling rejection. When dating, both men and women fear receiving no from the opposite sex because their self-worth feels in question.

Another factor in saying and hearing "no" relates to the movement from the parent/child to the adult paradigm. Here you recognize that you are not dependent on one or two people to meet your needs. When you receive a no it doesn't mean you lose hope of getting your needs met. It simply means you need to reach out to other sources—be persistent. When you accomplish this you have a newly developed self-concept model of an adult awareness, rather than the old parent/child model.

Lyn felt that she had run out of options for finding a husband who would accept her and her three children. She had had several relationships where men would soon lose interest in her when they found out she had a ready-made family. At first she felt rejected and thought her children were liabilities. As she continued doing her personal work she realized that, to be happy, she needed a partner who not only wanted to be a husband, but who really desired being part of a family. Shortly thereafter she met a man who had never had any children and was excited at the thought of becoming an integral part of her family.

It's nice to be reminded that God says no, too.

When you begin to unconditionally love others to the degree that they can say "no"—and unconditionally love yourself when you say "no"—you feel empowered. You now have a much larger container in which to live your life. How many times have you prayed for something and didn't receive what you asked for? If God can say no, certainly you can give yourself the license to say no and feel good about yourself.

Self-Validating

As you begin to accept a positive picture of yourself, your self-concept becomes more fluid because you see yourself differently. You can compliment yourself. Instead of thinking that you are arrogant or conceited because you think positively, you now realize that self-validation expands your healthy good feelings about yourself and strengthens your self-esteem.

You make the choice to begin self-validating.

Joy had a stuttering problem and was very nervous about entering a group. She had been brought up in an upper class New York environment where it wasn't "good form" to speak well of yourself. "Good form" was to say little or nothing about your accomplishments or good qualities. In that situation, you were simply to feel good about yourself because of your class and inherited wealth. However, this was not enough to comfort Joy or give her a sense of security. From the time she entered kindergarten till she graduated from high school she felt inferior to her peers. She seemed unable to do well scholastically or fit in socially which, of course, embarrassed her parents. She was afraid to speak up and voice her opinions. After months of saying nothing in the group, she realized she wasn't going to move forward unless she was able to voice her insecurities and validate her positive traits. The stuttering diminished when she started complimenting and validating—this allowed her to be comfortable enough to share her thoughts and feelings in a social setting. As Joy developed the inner voice of the good mother and the good father, she let go of the critical judgments of her parents.

Once you develop your capacity to self-validate, you are able to release old judgments and begin to feel more accepting and loving towards yourself. In other words, as you choose to listen to the voice of the internal good parents you hear less negativity, which allows you to spend less time in pain and more in self-love—positive self-regard then increases. Emotional changes get rooted into place through early conditioning. In order to live more fully in the present, you must release negative statements from the past and replace them with positive messages.

People want to see you at your best; they want to see you as beautiful, intelligent, creative capable, joyful and wise.

Not only does the active choice to self-validate, give you better feelings about yourself, you also discover that the more you compliment yourself, the more you attract people who compliment and validate you.

Contact vs. Content Relationships with Your Parents

Once you begin accepting all your new rights, letting go of the "be perfect script", saying and hearing no, and acknowledging your right to self-validate, you are prepared to distinguish between those parental relationships that are merely "contact" and those that have "content."

A "contact" relationship means you accept your parents as they are. You don't try to process anything with them and you don't attempt to change them. In this kind of relationship you are able to acknowledge their biological significance—they gave you life—and you are grateful for that. You release the expectation that your

parents "should" have been masters and accept instead that they (just like you) had to learn how to be parents.

Jordon had grown up in a Greek family where he watched his father yell and scream obscenities at his mother. Unfortunately, his father felt justified in this behavior because he had watched his parents behave in that same abusive manner. Now, as Jordon was planning to get married, he had a deep-rooted fear that he would behave toward his future wife the way his father had treated his mother. In his men's group he became consciously aware that he wanted to act differently toward his future wife. He wanted to speak to her respectively and end this ancestral pattern of verbal abuse and degradation. When he connected with his false feelings of superiority, Jordan was able to consciously make the necessary changes in his marriage. However, when he and his wife would go home for the holidays he found that he reverted to his old behavior of becoming distressed when witnessing the incessant arguments between his parents. At this point in his journey, Jordan realized his father was totally incapable of changing his behavior, that his father's words were automatic not unlike a tape player. Once he saw his father's predicament he was able to forgive him and let go of his old resentments. He could accept his father even if he couldn't accept his father's behavior. Therefore, he had a contact relationship with his father. He knew he couldn't change his father's behavior—he could only change his own view of him.

There is recognition that your journey entails learning what your parents didn't learn.

This process supports forgiveness and letting go of old resentments.

As you can see, it is easy to slip back into the Stage One feelings of victimization when you visit an old environment. One sign of having reached Stage Two is being able to separate the script that is communicated from the person communicating it. On the other hand, if you do have the good fortune to have a "content" relationship with a parent, it is possible to process the relationship in addition to bringing unconditional love to it. Processing change without judgment or condemnation is built on the fact that self-love knows how to ask for change.

"When I come to visit, I prefer staying at a motel and I will come home for meals."
"I would like you to know that my feelings were hurt when I told you about a big success. It seemed that everyone moved to the next subject without any acknowledgment of that success." "I was really hurt when you withheld the news that Dad was having surgery. I would appreciate, in the future, that you keep me informed about matters of illness or expected loss."

Many people try to process with their parents only to learn it isn't possible. It's helpful to let go of the attitude that your parents know your wishes without you voicing them. You can ask for the changes, although you have to be able to distinguish whether your parents can truly make them. It's important to consider whether your parents have the ability to stretch, how rigid their unconscious scripts might be, or how evolved they are. In Stage One you may feel that your parent's ability to change is a reflection on you. Stage Two brings the realization that this is more about them. If you find that it is not possible to overtly initiate positive change in relationships—whether with parents or others—it is valuable to realize that it may not be necessary.

Susan always complained that her mother interrupted her when she expressed a difference of opinion. No matter how often she tried to explain to her mother how important it was for her to accept their differences, her mother still continued to interrupt. After processing her frustration for several months, Susan realized she had reached the point where she could accept her mother's perspective and release the need to voice her differing opinion. Her self-esteem no longer depended on her mother's willingness to listen to her point of view or her mother's approval.

Change most often occurs as a result of your own shift of perspective. A neutral zone develops where there is mutual acceptance of the differences. Expectations that you and others should think and feel alike diminish.

Staying on Course

As you continue to develop a new positive self-concept you find that loving yourself brings loving people into your life. The more you respect yourself, the more you are attracted to those groups of people who want to embrace a positive self-concept. You observe how some of your old friends and associates may move out of your life because they may feel uncomfortable with all the changes you have made. You know that your relationships mirror what you believe about yourself. Every relationship in your life reflects your self-worth. This also holds true of your experiences in the world. Your life experiences manifest what you believe you deserve. You seek out learning environments that reinforce the true you.

It is here that you stretch, expand and grow through the choice of loving unconditionally.

Affirmations for Stage Two

Affirmations provide the language that fits the true you. Describing something is essential for manifesting. It is a way of programming the mind. You either give it a program of thought that supports you or you stay with the programming that demoralized and pulled you down. Affirmations are a powerful technique that:

- gives form to the new self-concept.
- allows you to practice speaking out loud the new wonderful truth about you.
- reinforces the new self-concept.
- replaces negative self-talk that keeps you stuck in the past.
- builds an aura of positive attraction.

The positive self-concept you develop enables you to declare what you want, whether you are experiencing it or not. You now have the confidence to persist with positive self-talk while releasing the negative—trusting that the process will lead you to experiencing what you verbalize, such as:

- I choose to love and accept myself unconditionally.
- I deserve to be happy.
- My life has value; I am worthy of love and respect.
- Just because I breathe, I am lovable.
- I accept the whole package.

- I am lovable with my strengths and weaknesses.
- I love and accept my body just the way it is; I am lovable just the way I am.
- I am patient and compassionate with others and myself.
- I surround myself with people who love and care about me.
- I am perfect just the way I am. I am intelligent, beautiful and trustworthy.
- I am strong, capable and a joy to be around.
- I am a powerful, loving, creative being.
- I accept myself whether I am succeeding or making a mistake.
- I release the need to judge, criticize and find fault with others and myself.
- I choose to support, validate and praise.

The Road Ahead

The shift from Stage Two to Stage Three is exciting and far from difficult. In fact you realize that you are expanding and enhancing what you are already living. Here in Stage Two you learned how to re-script internal messages that changed the way you felt about yourself. You may have found yourself going back and forth between stages. As you re-scripted your parental messages, you uncovered new pockets of pain. The difference was that you didn't feel like the victim; instead you wanted to acknowledge and express your feelings. In Stage Two, as you practiced self-validation, you gave yourself space to experiment and try new behaviors—like complimenting yourself. You are willing to look back at your history bank any time that facilitates empowering yourself to say "no."

As you move into Stage Three, you are ready to take control of your life, to plan and create your future. You feel secure enough to expand your horizons and worthy enough to ask for what you want. Your vision is able to project forward into time. You want to manifest your destiny. Be all that you can be. Do the things you have always wanted to do. Have the things you have always wanted to have.

As you head into Stage Three, you re-script specific messages so that you can affect a change in your outer world. Life is always a mirror of your thoughts—both conscious and unconscious. The outer world shows you what you feel you deserve. It shows the divergence between what you say and what you believe internally.

Stage Three is about manifesting a new relationship with the material world. It includes career, health, loving relationships and financial well being. Before you can have all four you must believe that you merit them, have faith that the universe will provide them, understand that there are no limitations and, finally, trust that the mind can create it all.

Questions to Contemplate

- What were the conditions you were taught for gaining love and approval?
- Do you feel lovable when you say "no?"
- Is it harder to hear or say "no?"
- What messages did your parents give you that supported positive self-esteem?
- What messages diminished your self-esteem?

Stage 3

Manifesting What You Want

You become the creator of your life.

In this stage, we cover Letting Go of Poverty Scripts and Programming, Using The Creative Power of The Mind, Affirmations: Your Words of Power, and Manifesting Your Hearts Desires and Dreams.

The View From Here

As you enter the third stage of the spiritual journey, you have a positive self-regard and a conviction that you have a right to be happy and deserve to be prosperous. Now you learn the mental laws and principles for creating your deepest wishes and desires. You discover that if you can envision something, think it, and mentally accept it as a possibility, then you can create it. You have no

You now exercise the creative power of your mind.

doubt that you are able to manifest abundant good in your daily life. You write out your goals and objectives, visualize the future you desire, and use positive affirmations to expand your field of radiation and attraction. As you get focused and specific about what you want, you manifest your goals and dreams. Manifestation includes not only financial and material success but also experiencing loving relationships, peace of mind, and good health.

In discovering the creative power of the mind, you realize that the universe is generous and abundant and that your mind is unlimited in its ability to create. However, you can only manifest what you consciously or unconsciously believe you deserve. This may mean that you need to identify and let go of any scripts or programs that would make you feel undeserving or guilty about experiencing the abundant life that you are capable of creating.

> **"The world is my playground —a laboratory for discovering and experiencing the creator in me."**

The Transition from Stage Two to Stage Three

When you have made the shift from Stage Two to Stage Three, you have developed enough of a positive self-regard and self-esteem that you can truly believe you are worthy enough to experience prosperity. In Stage One, you created a vacuum where you released the negative scripts and emotions that kept you stuck in your past hurts and resentments.

In Stage Two, you created a new self-concept that supported your belief that you deserved unlimited good in your life. You survived enlightenment through pain; you went from being a victim, blaming yourself, others and circumstances—to taking responsibility for your life and actions. You have become the parent you have always wanted. You know how to listen to your needs and to forgive yourself and others for their ignorance as a cause of your suffering and pain. You are no longer caught up in the melodramas of the past or in the unconsciousness of denial. Now, you know you can nurture and support yourself and surround yourself with people who love and care about you.

In Stage Two, you also moved out of the past and its control over your feelings and emotions into the freedom of the present. You dismantled the old self-concept you inherited from parents and replaced it with a new positive self-regard. You let go of the "be perfect" script and were willing to try new things, even if you couldn't get it right the first time you tried. You were willing to learn from your mistakes rather than reject yourself; self-correction was embraced. You discovered the more you loved and nurtured yourself, the more you brought into your life loving and nurturing people. You learned that you could choose to love yourself unconditionally—to accept all your strengths and weaknesses.

Now, in Stage Three, you find for the first time that the energy you used to validate and love yourself in Stage Two can open your awareness and expand your horizons to include the future. You have energy at your disposal to think beyond the present moment—to create the future. You synthesize your values and views of society and discover the things you "buy into." You are here to learn that being a creator of positive outcomes is an essential part of your growth on your journey. This is where you learn the relationship between thought and manifestation.

You are excited by the prospects ahead.

You are now learning how to manifest everything you desire on the physical plane. You are learning that you have the potential to manifest your dreams—to make them a reality in this physical world. You are a creator and manifestor and here to turn the energy of your mind into material manifestation. In Stages One and Two, you either did not have the belief in yourself that you deserved happiness, success and plenty—or you were wrapped up in your dramas of pain and unhappiness. You were in a fog where your vision was blinded by the issues of emotional survival, the limitations of your history and the limiting scripts you had learned from the past. After all, you told yourself good luck couldn't happen to anyone that had a run of bad breaks. Fortunately, the work you have done in enlightenment through pain and building a positive self-concept prepared you for a different response.

Creating Your Future

In Stage Three, you mobilize the powerful potential of your mind to create what you genuinely desire and want. The energy gained from releasing the past and believing in your own self-worth makes it possible to manifest goals, roles, health, happiness, success and money.

The future is created through thought; the future is the outcome of your thoughts.

All the experiences and growth to this point have changed something very fundamental inside of you. You are no longer being reactive or passively accepting what comes your way. Now it is time to create what you genuinely want and desire—to choose in the present the outcomes you desire. If you do not affirm what you want in the present, you won't have it in the future. You will simply experience the outcome of your old thoughts and beliefs. You must affirm, in the present, a future outcome before you can manifest a new result. Thought precedes manifestation.

The Lay of the Land

Phyllis' Stage Three Experience

In 1981, while living in Sarasota, Florida, Phyllis began reading *The Dynamic Laws of Prosperity*[1] by Catherine Ponder. At the time, she lived a very modest lifestyle and was in an unhappy marriage going nowhere. She had a small private practice and very little peace of mind. During the day, she did therapy in her office, and at night she slept on an air mattress on the floor. She did not have a kitchen. She ate all her meals at a Cuban restaurant. She owned few physical possessions, and had no savings or retirement account. Her assets included her creativity, enormous sensitivity and empathy, contacts with the New Age community, and the freedom to choose how she spent her time. She never worked for an agency and was always self-employed. She could choose when she wanted to work and come and go as she pleased. She spent a lot of time walking on the beach.

You have personally accomplished much to arrive at this point in the journey.

When she came across *The Dynamic Laws of Prosperity*, she had very little experience with money or planning her life. She had grown up in a middle-class family where she was an only child and amply provided for. Upon graduating from Boston University, she got married. The picture she had for herself was that there would always be someone to take care of her—that she could live day-by-day, freely expressing. She began her career in the performing arts as a professional artist. Later, she majored in religion as an undergraduate and finally became a psychotherapist after she received her Ph.D. in psychology. However, throughout all of this, she never planned for the future; she just seemed to fall into relationships and situations as they presented themselves and responded to what was offered.

Fortunately, when she encountered these teachings, she was ready to learn how to achieve financial prosperity and success and was eager to plan her future the way she wanted it. She was no longer willing to depend on persons and conditions outside. For the first time in her life, she wanted to take the reins of her life and gallop into a positive future, which she had control over—one she had planned.

Over the next few years, as Phyllis applied these mental laws and principles, she made several internal and external changes. She left her marriage and moved to New Mexico. She created a large vacuum and was starting over again. She had no one to turn to or depend on. She had to find money, clients, a home, friends, a personal relationship and the source and the power to manifest what she needed. Every morning she would awake around five. She would either drift into a floating anxiety or she would turn the light on, get out of bed and begin saying affirmations out loud. It was the process that had supported her moving across the country and leaving her marriage. She would begin by affirming there was a plan for her life and that it included happiness, success and financial prosperity. As she tapped into her deepest desires, she wrote out her goals with detailed timelines and descriptions.

She found that she began attracting people and opportunities for a successful practice, a significant increase in earning power, and a loving and supportive relationship. During that period, each time she had a doubt or a negative thought she would not repress or ignore it, rather she would replace it with a positive affirmation. She persisted until she had the increase she'd affirmed. In the next five years, she quadrupled her income. It all began with the belief that the source of her success was within, as well as in the attitudes and thoughts she chose to give time and energy to.

She spent many evenings sitting alone creating a wheel of fortune, cutting out pictures from magazines, organizing and pasting them on poster board, creating a visual picture of what she desired in life. At one point, she made a wheel of fortune with a picture of a couple traveling on safari. There were large bills of play money and a flashy red Miata sports car in front of a beautiful patio home. Six months later, when her future husband turned up in his white Fiat convertible with the top down, she smiled a knowing smile. A year and a half later, when they were happily married, they went on her very first cruise in the Aegean Sea, taking along her daughters.

Manifesting Results in the First Curriculum

Now, in Stage Three, you engage your will to assert positively your dreams and wishes for material success and happiness. You continually build your self-confidence and determination by persisting to affirm what you want and to bring it to fruition. You believe in the power of your thoughts and that you can be the master of your destiny. You choose your thoughts; therefore you can choose the outcomes you desire.

Your energy is boundless.

Each day is an opportunity to advance, to achieve, and to experience greater abundance and success in your life. If you think it, you know you can create it. You are the author of your life; your ego is strong and feels confident and focused; it believes that it can produce what it desires. Your mind is brimming with ideas, the wheels are churning, and you bubble over with enthusiasm and delight. Your mind is cooking with possibilities; night and day you have boundless energy; and, as you achieve your goals, your

You are ready to step up to the plate, to get on base, to hit a single, double, even a home run with the bases loaded.

confidence and excitement for life grows. You can't wait to write out your goals and envision your future. You are eager to affirm the good you want; you devote your time and energy daily to reviewing and revising your goals, thinking and re-thinking what you desire to achieve. Life is good, very good indeed.

You have discovered the secret of success. It's all within the power of your mind to generate the thoughts and ideas that can construct your reality as you wish it to be; you are like a genie with an Aladdin's lamp. You can wish it, conceive it and make it happen. You no longer doubt that you deserve to be wealthy. You feel that you were born to be happy and have a right to claim your happiness now. You embrace and accept the good life, financial prosperity, career success, personal happiness and material comforts and toys. Your five senses are alive and stimulated. You feel that you are an active player in the world of your life. Your lifestyle sizzles with the anticipation and achievement of your goals. You are in the driver's seat, confident that you can get any place you desire; a red light or flat tire are just momentary stops. You are not afraid of life, rather you are an active participant ready and eager to engage and play the game.

You love your life and feel in control.

It is important to remember that none of the stages happen overnight—it is a process of active engagement. It is not just a way of thinking and saying you understand. It is a way of living an organic process that depends on the amount of time, attention, and your willingness to devote to the journey, your desire to grow and move forward.

Guidelines for Stage Three

The Adult Consciousness

When you come into Stage Three, it is your adult, not the child or the parent, who is going to create on the physical, emotional, and mental levels your goals and dreams. The child can't do it. The child belongs in Stages One and Two.

When you were in enlightenment through pain and building your positive self-esteem, the child had the starring role and took center stage. The journey was about healing, re-parenting, and building positive good feelings about self. In Stage Three, the adult has the starring role; the adult has access to the principles of manifestation and has the will to persist and succeed. "I am the creator and generator of my life."[2]

The child can't implement on the physical level.

As the adult, you are no longer in the dependent role of a child, dependent on one or two people to take care of your needs and be the singular source of your happiness. You are no longer confined to the "house of your parents"—physically, psychologically or emotionally. Instead, the adult mind connects you to unlimited channels that can fulfill your needs. Now, you can connect with many sources, people, opportunities and circumstances.

The adult mind has access to the wisdom, the universal laws, principles and the ability to think. Therefore, in Stages One and Two you set the foundation for the adult to come on stage. The adult was building and developing when you were learning how to work enlightenment through pain. Your adult was there—supporting the new self-concept. It is in Stage Three, as an adult, that you move out

The world is your new home, workplace and playground.

of the dependency of the child-parent mode to not only being able to take care of your basic needs, but also to where you are now able to create a dynamic and inspiring life.

Now, in Stage Three, you discover yourself as a creator. Your mind is the link between thought and supply. It changes attitudes about what is possible for you mentally, accepting the possibility of something better for yourself. The adult aligns with the intuitive mind and loves the best and highest in life. You change your experience of the world by changing your mental perspective. You believe there is a plan and purpose for your life. Part of your self-concept includes prosperity and an abundance of good. You have found the point of power within you.

Aspects of the Adult Mind

The adult mind has mental control: if I have control over my thoughts, I have control over my life. In enlightenment through pain, it was nearly impossible to have this kind of mental control. Your emotions were volatile and unstable; you were so reactive that you couldn't focus long enough to think beyond the moment of your immediate pain and discomfort. When building your positive self-concept, you began to gain more control over your thoughts in the present. You learned to choose your self-talk and thereby affect your feelings of well being and self-worth.

The adult has the vision to realize a future dream before it is actualized.

In Stage Three, the adult has the ability to conceive in advance what it wants before it manifests. This is unlike the experience in enlightenment through pain where there was little hope or future, and you could barely keep your head above water—you felt the only choice you had was fight, freeze or flight. Now, in Stage Three, your adult has a map, timelines, the discipline, persistence, and determination to reach its goal. The use of the will predominates.

Master Plan

The adult knows that life has order and purpose; there is a Master Plan. Life isn't simply a random expression of events, over which you have little or no say or control. The adult believes there is a greater overarching plan for life and that this plan includes past, present and future. The adult has access to this Master Plan and is no longer stuck in day-to-day activities and routines, existing and not joyously living life.

In Stage Three, the focus of this Master Plan is about successfully creating and manifesting the dreams and expectations of the first curriculum: financial and material wealth, career success, a happy marriage, loving healthy family, and a lifestyle that includes vacations, travel, hobbies and adult toys. The Master Plan focuses on the self as creator and manifestor, personally satisfying all desires.

Later in the second curriculum, during Stage Five, the Master Plan will expand its focus to community and service and be more outward directed to the needs of the planet. But now, in Stage Three, the adult learns how to be in charge of his/her personal existence before having the control and experience to positively affect a larger group or community mission.

Stage Three Work

Principle—Thought Is Creative

As I change my thoughts, I change my world. As I improve my thoughts, I improve my world. As I transform my thoughts, I transform my world.[3] *As I tap into the adult mindset, I can mentally accept the possibility of something better for me. As I open up my mind to prosperity and abundance, I begin to attract the ideas, opportunities, events, and people who can help me succeed and achieve material wealth. As I open my mind to prosperity, as I dwell upon thoughts of plenty, as I begin to picture the desires of my heart, as I write out my goals, I build a field of mental attraction that draws the very things I say I want. If I think it, I can create it. First, I mentally focus on my wants, through a thought, through an image, through an affirmation, through a written goal—and thereby attract it to me.*

Principle—Thought and Manifestation Are All One and the Same Energy

Science continues to demonstrate that matter and energy are interchangeable.

Albert Einstein with $E=mc^2$ opened the door to the construct that energy can be converted into matter and vice versa. In Stage Three, you are here to learn how the transfer of energy operates in your life. As you have been paying close attention to your own life with all its daily changes, you are aware that the formed and the unformed worlds come from the same source. Living with increasing conscious awareness reveals that the visible and invisible realms are relative.

For almost everyone, a solid object is real, while thoughts are considered less real. Now you begin to learn that thoughts and solid objects are all one and the same energy. Your thoughts can immediately create something on the mental plane; the physical manifestation takes longer. In either dimension, it is still all the same energy.

When Kathy was planning her wedding at the home of a friend, she was able to visualize the entire wedding in her mind. She saw everything she wanted: the food, how she would be dressed, where it would take place, the ceremony and the people. She could picture it and even feel the good feelings that went along with the experience. However, on the days preceding the wedding, as well as the wedding day itself, implementing all the details on the physical level took a lot more time and effort.

Principle—Field of Unlimited Potential

You live in a field of unlimited potential; the energy for creation is unlimited; your job is to create the mental concepts for what you want to manifest on the material plane in this physical world. As you take this energy, which is undefined and amorphous, and begin to organize and define it, you manifest your reality.

Principle—Radiation and Attraction

Thought is magnetic:

I am an irresistible magnet, with the power to attract unto myself everything I genuinely desire, according to the thoughts, feelings and mental pictures I constantly entertain and radiate. I am the center of my universe. I have the power to create whatever I wish. I attract whatever I radiate. I attract whatever I mentally choose and accept.[5]

Your thoughts either attract or repel the good you say you want. The world around you is a mirror of your thoughts. You may say, "Why is there so much unhappiness, or lack, or failure? I work so hard, put out all this effort, and have so little to show for it." Your attitude affects your experience. Your life is always a mirror of your thinking, not only what you are consciously thinking, but also more importantly what your unconscious believes and thinks. Your experience doesn't only mirror your conscious thoughts, but your unconscious thoughts as well.

Whenever there seems to be a division between what you outwardly say you want and have, you know there must be a contrary unconscious thought or feeling. At this point in the journey, your awareness of your thoughts is heightened. You take responsibility to identify the script that is blocking the field of attraction.

Poverty Scripts and Programming

Many of you grew up believing that money was "the root of all evil" or that people who have money can't be spiritual. Some hide their success or downplay their net worth. They are afraid of the envy and jealousy that wealth evokes in others. When you reach Stage Three, you begin to understand that God, the Creator, isn't a being outside and separate from you. Rather, in your adult consciousness, you are the Mind of God. You are the creator and manifestor of your life. You have learned the principles of

You may feel guilty or think it unfair that some people have and others don't.

creation and now can convert energy into matter through the power of your mind.

Money is nothing more than a symbol of the unlimited field of energy, which is at the disposal for everyone. Believe it, and you can apply these mental principles of creation. When comparisons are made between the rich and the poor, the haves and have nots, what separates them is not the labels and the conditions but the consciousness that has created them. Everyone evolves stage-by-stage, one step at a time.

Tithing

Giving a tenth of what you earn to the source of your spiritual power increases your field of attraction. Tithing was a thoroughly new concept for Bruce. The thought that giving could make him rich was something he hadn't really considered before. Since he was still in a learning mode and experiencing some career success, he wanted to practice what he had been taught about tithing.

He decided to try it and tithe his tenth with the expectation of a hundred-fold return. His first experience was in a Unity Church. He had gone to the Midwest and had earned more in one week than he had earned in that entire month. When he stood up to give, he felt his heart burst open and an incredible feeling of joy well up inside of him. In that moment, he knew he wanted to feel that wonderful, exhilarating feeling of giving—again and again. He vowed to give ten times as much. Over the next 15 years he did exactly that and experienced a 100-fold return.

You can increase your field of attraction by tithing.

In Stage Three, the experience of being a giver is incredibly inspiring and exciting. It often alleviates the guilt that you might have too much and that others are starving with little or no material wealth.

Principle—Creating a Vacuum—Release Makes You Magnetic

Nature abhors a vacuum. Therefore, you must create a space for the new you want by letting go of the old that no longer serves. In Stage Three, release makes you magnetic to your highest good; it removes emotional blocks and barriers that make you less magnetic to attracting your heart's desires. Release is about letting go of your attachment to things, places and persons that no longer support your goals, dreams and desires. What you project is what you attract. When you let go, you send out a clear signal that you are ready to receive the good you say you want. The quicker you let go, the more magnetic you become. In the past, release was often associated with loss, losing something, or experiencing lack. Often because of fear of loss, you held on to situations and conditions which probably met only a portion of your needs. You might have believed that having half a loaf is better than having nothing at all.

If you hang on to what you don't want, how can you attract what you do want?

Now, in Stage Three, letting go is an active, conscious choice. It is about being really clear about your priorities—about what you truly want and don't want. It is a fearless statement to the world about who you are, what you are about, and what you will and won't accept for yourself. Release is making room, creating a larger space for good to come into your life.

Let go of the lesser to attract the greater.

Releasing on the Physical Level

Only hold on to those things that are unequivocally positive and empowering.

Releasing must begin on the physical level. In this world, you experience the relationship between mind and matter. Your goal is to master the art of manifesting what you want on the material level. This is something you are here to learn, not minimize or ignore. It is part of your spiritual journey. For example, you could dispose of old papers, books, clothes, furniture and physical possessions that you truly no longer want in your life.

Often, the emotional is tied to the physical as well. Old memories, associations, melancholy, and nostalgia may attach you to things that no longer represent who you are in the present and where you want to go in the future. The decision to let go of physical objects facilitates the process of getting rid of emotional and mental baggage. Make everything in your life support your new consciousness; if it doesn't make you glow, it goes. Remember you want to glow and be magnetic to your good.

When Gloria moved from Cincinnati to Sarasota, she released all her books on philosophy that she had used in graduate school. She was never going to use those books again. She was going to a spiritual ashram. Her mind was elsewhere. She released hundreds of books because she didn't want to carry that energy forward with her—she was open to new schools of learning.

Memories Attached to Physical Objects

As you are going through the process of letting go, remember that all physical objects absorb the energy of the time in which you lived and used them. They've absorbed your depression, your fights with your spouse, your sadness, and your disappointments.

Nathan was terribly distressed. When he was driving home late one night after seeing a play, he had a horrible experience: a drunk committed suicide by throwing himself in front of his car. A year later, when Nathan was still having terrible dreams about the experience, he mentioned to his counselor that whenever he rode in the car, he thought about how the man's body brushed him through the sunroof. "You mean to tell me that you still drive the same car?" said the astonished counselor. "Sell it immediately!" the counselor advised. Thereafter, the nightmares stopped.

Nearly everyone has the tendency to want to take things from one environment into another. It seems natural to want to be reminded of the past. If the object carries total positive associations, that's fine. If, however, it keeps you attached to memories that are not helpful to the process of creating a new vision—let them go.

After a divorce, you want to let go of everything that is associated with the bedroom—the bed and bedding—because you don't want to carry forward those old, painful memories and associations. You want to create a vacuum to attract a new significant and intimate relationship.

It is equally significant to bring order into your life to prepare for the arrival of the new. Getting organized is helpful—updating, reviewing, and organizing records, letters, business files—so that everything you regularly come in contact with has been looked through, released, and put in order. It is also necessary to make sure there isn't any unfinished business that will appear from the past to confuse or muddy your magnetic field of attraction.

If you release something, something equal or better will replace it.

A business friend, Georgia, was complaining that she was low on funds. She discovered she had not sent out her billing for several thousand dollars of past consulting work. Before she could attract new work and money, she had to set up a systematic billing system and send out the past-due bills. Once that was accomplished, her receivables were cleared and new business started to flow.

Releasing on the Emotional Level

The ability to forgive and release allows love to radiate, and that's the universal energy for attraction. Every negative thought you have blocks the goodness that is waiting for you. To become a positive field of attraction, you have to forgive and let go. You cannot afford the luxury of a negative thought.[6] Putting out the message that nothing can be withheld from you is necessary. What is genuinely yours can never be taken from you. If a relationship no longer supports your happiness, if your needs are not being met, if you have outgrown a relationship, taken different paths or gone in opposite directions, let it go. By letting go of a dissatisfying relationship, you open your mind and heart to a new relationship that is fulfilling.

> **Your will is pointed upward and forward.**

The work you did in enlightenment through pain supports your ability to become the good parent who acknowledged and responded to your needs. You realized, through the act of forgiveness, that you could let go of the past so that your needs could be met in the present. By letting go of the anger and hurt in Stage One, you moved into Stage Two and were able to receive the unconditional love you deserved.

Now, in Stage Three, when you are caught up in reactive emotions, such as feelings of disappointment and resentment, you have the will and mental fortitude to convert the negative into a positive. You practiced this in Stages One and Two, and now your will to succeed is stronger than the pull of your upset. You now want to convert your initial feelings of hurt and anger into an assertive, proactive response.

Rather than recycling negative feelings over and over, release them. Identify either what you need to self-correct or learn and move forward to face the future. Suppose you were asked to leave a job. Instead of holding on to resentment, feelings of unfairness, or picturing yourself as a victim of circumstances, it would be best to mobilize your mental energy to visualize a job equal to or better than what you had. The more quickly you release and forgive, the more magnetic your field of attraction becomes and the sooner you will attract a new job opportunity.

Basic Methods of Manifesting

Affirmations

To "affirm" means to make firm the good you want in your life. As discussed before, an affirmation is a statement of positive intent—an assertion about your future good. *"I love the highest and best in life, and I attract the highest and best in life to me now."*[7] Affirmations replace the old scripts with positive statements of confidence and success. *"I am aligned with the upward, progressive movement of life; the mark of success is now upon me."*[8] As affirmations are repeated, they create a magnetic field of attraction. The spoken word literally changes the auric field and speeds up the process of achieving your goals. *"My words have prospering power now".* [9]

You awake each day and feel grateful.

Affirmations build your positive self-concept so that you believe you have the right to be happy and deserve an abundant life. You are eager to start the day. The thought of doing what you love brings a surge of energy to your body. *"Today and every day I expect the best. Wonderful things are happening to me now!"*[10]

Using affirmations opens your mind to prosperity and accelerates the good to appear. You are now creating new scripting. The internalization of ideas is crucial to the organic process. You need to restructure your mental framework in order to accept these new ideas and possibilities. *"I am now shown new ways of living, new methods of growth. I am not confined to the ways and methods of the past."*[11]

In any situation, you can ask yourself, *"Am I in emotional upset?" Does this call for a release or forgiveness affirmation? "I forgive myself and others."*[12] Does my self-esteem and confidence need a boost in the present? Does this call for a confidence affirmation? *"Nothing is too good to be true."*[13] Do I want to plan for the future and project my field of radiation to attract wealth and success? Does this call for a prosperity affirmation? *"I dare to prosper."*[14]

Therefore, affirmations for Stage Three help you focus on prosperity and build your field of radiation—moving you from being a 75-watt bulb to being a 150-watt bulb. These affirmations attract material wealth, build self-confidence for expansion in your career and broaden your experience of life.

Nothing in the world can take the place of persistence and determination. *Don't get discouraged. Imagine a bucket, where one affirmation is only a drop—how many drops does it take to fill the bucket?* [15]

Affirmations for Stage Three

- If I can think it, I can create it.
- I desire and attract the best in every aspect of my life.
- I am open to receive the vast wealth the universe has for me.
- I love the work I do, and I am richly rewarded for it.
- I have a large, steady financial income now.
- Every day and in every way, things are getting better and better for me.

Goal Setting

It's important to write down your goals. A goal is not, "I want to be rich" or "I want to be famous." Those are dreams. They are too vague. If you can't describe it or attach a number to it, it's a wish, not a goal. Goals require deadlines. This can be flexible—you don't abandon a worthwhile goal simply because you didn't achieve it by a specific date. It is important that you project an outcome so that the unconscious mobilizes your internal forces.

Get definite about what you want.

A recent study was designed to see how many graduates were achieving their goals ten years after graduation. Incredibly, 83 percent had no goals at all. Fourteen percent claimed to have specific goals but had not written them down. This group's average income was three times greater than the 83 percent group. More to the point, the remaining three percent, who had written goals, were earning ten times as much as the 83 percent group.

Besides writing your goals on paper, it is also key that you read, review, and revise them daily so that the unconscious mind can fully integrate their meaning.

Giving thanks in anticipation of good happening is essential. This way you are claiming in the present future good, defining it the way you want it to actualize. By anticipating your good, you accelerate good coming to you. If perhaps there is a consulting contract you want to secure, an expression of gratitude in the present supports the attainment of your goal. Giving thanks in advance helps this contract to be consummated.

Don't forget to give yourself credit when you have achieved a goal.

In Stage Three, you also have the opportunity to jointly set goals in your marriage or partnership. Together, get definite about the future. It may be best to create a one-, two-, three- and four-year plan. First, focus on short-term goals and create a monthly budget. Next, discuss long-term goals and create a schedule for financial investment and saving. Also, make some decisions regarding vacations and planning for your children's higher education.

When you are definite about your goals, it is meaningful to make sure that they are your goals not what others expect or don't expect, or think you should or shouldn't have. When you get in touch with your deepest heartfelt desires, you are closest to the author and creator of this magnificent universe, and therefore, you are the closest to the essence of yourself—the creator and manifestor.

Visualization

When you use the imaging power of the mind, you put your imagination to work. As you mentally picture the success, wealth, and happiness you want, your mind will prepare for this to happen.

One way to visualize would be to create a collage of what you want by cutting out pictures from magazines and assembling them on a poster board. By looking at it often, your conscious and unconscious mind is reminded of what you desire. You might want to sell a house for a certain amount of money. Take a picture of that house and place a sold sign over it with the price you want. Put it in a prominent place so that you can see it frequently. If you are looking to create a happy relationship, paste a happy photograph of yourself onto a poster board, then add images and words of interactions that are loving and intimate.

Whatever the mind is taught to expect, it will manifest.

The second way is to mentally visualize with your eyes closed, in a relaxed state, an image of what you want. It is as if you have a movie screen in your mind where you can project your desired picture. Joe wanted a summer apartment at the ocean, directly on the beach so that he could have an unobstructed view. He visualized himself standing, looking out of the living room window directly at the ocean. He could hear the waves crash, smell the ocean air and see people walking along the beach. A week later, when he began looking in earnest and after only two rejections, he found the house just as he had envisioned it.

These pictures and images you create mentally increase self-confidence and expand your field of radiation. They make you magnetic and accelerate you manifesting results.

Staying on Course

In Stage Three, you come to believe you are the architect of your life. If something isn't right, it can be fixed. There may be some of you who have been very successful at manifesting in a single dimension—let's say in the area of material wealth—but find the rest of your life is less than happy. This may mean that you have issues that haven't been resolved, issues impairing your abilities to manifest. At this juncture, you may find yourself returning to earlier stages. For instance, perhaps you find that you are in pain similar to Stage One and need to review your history bank again. If you are in need of boosting your confidence, you can return to Stage Two and strengthen your self-esteem. If you need a vision for projecting your goals forward into the future, you may need to continue working Stage Three.

Each step of the journey builds upon the last.

Keep in mind that change is constant and you need to be psychologically prepared to be open and affirming toward doing the work. It's important to have the ability to address issues as they naturally emerge in your life, therefore it helps to develop the flexibility to move in and out of any stage. You might even find yourself working all three stages at once, which can be challenging. When you master certain lessons, you feel more in control of your life—like accepting yourself unconditionally. This can give you access to an unlimited supply of energy that can accelerate your growth. This is the time when you become capable of being able to discriminate whether you are in the past, the present or the future and where you need to focus your time and attention.

Staying on course is not necessarily a linear progression.

When you are working in Stage Three, and not manifesting abundant good, you know that the conscious and unconscious are not in tune. Health, peace, love and prosperity are what you desire, not just one part of the package. Without harmony in all areas, there could be a significant amount of pain and unhappiness. You manifest what you know in both your conscious and unconscious existence. Your view of the world is a picture of what you feel you deserve. The reality around you reveals with inescapable honesty what you are emotionally capable of accepting.

Now you find yourself approaching the end of the first curriculum, where you will want to recapitulate the past by not only looking back and focusing on your childhood, but by evaluating what you learned and gained from your adult life experience.

You are at the bridge to transition from the first curriculum into the second. You are at a major critical choice point: you can remain in the first curriculum, doing your work, or, if you choose, you can enter and start a new curriculum.

As you come to the bridge, you are leaving one territory, one state of consciousness, one view of your life and what it is about.

The Road Ahead

Stage Three marks the conclusion of the first curriculum. You have accomplished much. You have evaluated your history bank, developed self-esteem, and have manifested in the world. The second curriculum brings an entirely new set of issues such as defining the meaning and purpose of the rest of your life, asking the big questions, and discovering how you can co-create in community.

However, before you can address the second curriculum, you first enter Stage Four, where you will be re-evaluating what you learned from the first curriculum, how it worked or didn't work for you, what you accomplished and what you ignored or overlooked. You are ready to go through a major life review—realizing that the principles and criteria you learned in the first curriculum are not necessarily transferable to the second. In fact, you may or may not be aware that you have the opportunity to create a second curriculum. You may not know what is ahead of you—you do know that you can't repeat what you have already lived out. You also have a sense of adventure in discovering what will be dynamic and passionate for your future. This time, though, you are not starting from scratch as an infant—you have experience and learning behind you

Now you are entering the heart of the journey. It is here that you meet the parts of your personality that have been dormant, unknown or repressed. You face the challenge of recognizing your shadow self—the parts of you that haven't been expressed because they didn't support your self-image of success or financial prosperity. Suddenly, you have questions that can't be answered. You feel uncertain, less black and white, and assuredly far less definite. In fact, you may find that the answers you seek aren't available in the outer world. It becomes clear that this is the time when you have to search inside for inner guidance and direction. Your life as you have known it feels like it is coming to close. The future is an open door. This is where you ask the questions, "Is there more than what I know and have experienced? Can I evolve beyond what I've already mastered? Is this all there is?"

Questions to Contemplate

- If your world is a reflection of your thoughts, what feedback is your world giving you about your thinking?
- What scripts did you learn that might have made you feel guilty about money, implying that money was the root of all evil and that poverty was a virtue?
- What are you willing to release to create the vacuum that will make you more magnetic to your good?
- Without any limitations such as judgments from outside sources, how might your goals have been different for the first curriculum?

End Notes

[1-15] *The Dynamic Laws Of Prosperity* by Catherine Ponder.

Stage 4

Bridging the Gap Between Past & Future

To move forward you must build a bridge between your past and future.

In this stage, we cover A Major Life Review, Embracing Your Shadow, Letting Go of What No Longer Serves You, and Taking the Best from the Past.

The View From Here

As you enter Stage Four, you feel as if you have finished an enormous work. It's as if you have climbed a great mountain. Some of you may have even reached the top, the summit. As you stand back and review all that you have achieved, you feel proud of your efforts and your accomplishments—you have met the challenges.

At this moment, as you stand on top of the mountain and review your life, you are aware that you traveled through infancy, early childhood, pre-school, grade school, puberty, adolescence and high school. The late teens and early 20s are defined by issues of occupational choices and additional schooling whereas; developmental milestones of the 20s, 30s and 40s may involve dating, marriage, children, education, career, and financial security. You've established your roles as son or daughter, brother or sister, acquaintance, friend, lover, student, worker, entrepreneur, husband, wife, significant other and parent.

During these years, many of you defined yourself through the predetermined structure that society or your parents built. Now you are experiencing a state of ambivalence where everything appears to be gray and nothing is just black or white—everything is both/and. You feel you can't use the same curriculum for the future because the present is too full of change and feels off center.

In Stage Four, you find you have to work both the past and present because so much is changing in your life. You need to recapitulate the past before projecting into the future. You conclude that you can't use previous models for the rest of your life, which is one of the predicaments of Stage Four. The time has come to identify the jewels/wisdom of the past so that you know what to carry forward. It is here that you are confronted with parts of the first curriculum that you didn't complete satisfactorily. You realize that, before you can move forward and make the connection to your soul and inner guidance system, you must first complete the work of the first curriculum. Now, in Stage Four, you are confronted both by an ending and a beginning.

Bob had always done what he was told and was successful doing so. He went to the prep school his parents selected; he went to college where all the men in his family had attended; and he went to the same medical school—all the while assured of success, money and prestige. Now, in his mid-30s, when out of medical school and working a couple years, he felt a lack of enthusiasm about performing surgeries every day. He knew his heart was not in it. He began questioning why he had chosen medicine. At age 20, there was never a doubt in his mind. Now, looking back, he wondered if it was really what he wanted or was it nothing more than an expectation. As the feeling of resistance grew, he stepped out of character and spontaneously signed up for an African safari.

For two weeks he was totally disconnected from his family, work, peers and daily routine. When Bob returned, he began questioning his entire life. He had never questioned who he married, how many children he should have or even if he should have children, where he should live, what profession he should pursue, or how much income he should earn. This had all been planned for him—long before he had taken his first breath. His entire life, Bob had conscientiously followed a script without resistance. When he was younger it seemed logical, the right thing to do. By all outward standards, he was a success.

Now, he was feeling a void in the pit of his stomach, a gnawing feeling that wouldn't go away—as if something was missing. He was no longer certain that he was doing what he genuinely wanted to do or if he was simply living out his family's dream of success. To explore his feelings and question every aspect of his life, he joined a group where he received support to further ask life-changing questions.

You knew you could get by on your strengths and you avoided areas of discomfort.

As you begin to look back, you can see where you made compromises, left parts of yourself behind, perhaps lived out other's dreams and expectations, or avoided dealing with parts of self that were weaknesses and not strengths. It is now, in Stage Four, that you begin to face your shadow—which is the largest piece of work you will have to address in building your bridge to your second curriculum. Your goal is to realize and begin to live out possibilities and dreams that didn't have expression before.

In this portion of the journey, you may feel like you are experiencing the discomfort of being an adolescent again. You know intellectually that you have everything you wanted. For some unexplained reason, having everything doesn't seem to matter anymore. You watch your spouse, recognizing little habits you've always told yourself were endearing twitches and are now horrified to find yourself wondering if you must stay with this person for the rest of your life. You feel impatient and restless. Even though these aren't unfamiliar feelings, they seem different this time. They feel more intense, more real, and more serious. You feel that if you continue to give in to the "shoulds," you'll die inside. It appears that the road ahead has two forks, neither of which looks particularly appealing. You can't keep doing what you've been doing because you begin to think you're getting old, not that you're losing your capacity—quite the contrary, you've never been better at what you do.

Changes that occur at this time in a life span are revolutionary.

This dissatisfaction that emerges in Stage Four signals a life change that is completely transformational, emotional in its intensity, and can be extremely tumultuous. It follows the traditional dramatic arc of defining something to be desired, meeting setbacks, and finding ways through them to realize an accomplishment. Boy meets girl, boy loses girl, and boy gets girl, as the usual plot of a movie love story is summarized. Now, in Stage Four, you discover that you don't want to be what you've been any more. Who are you then?

The work you did in Stages One, Two and Three feels like a complete life.

For the first time in your life, you realize that learning comes from internal forces, not external ones. The dictates of others—parents, family, school, marital expectations, the needs of dependents, the work world—have been for the most part resolved or satisfied. There's enough money, thanks to all that manifesting in Stage Three, and the challenge of goal setting and goal meeting feels a bit flat. The usual patterns—everything that has worked so well, all the challenges that were addressed and met—no longer hold any appeal. And, suddenly, long-forgotten aspects of the self show signs of re-emerging.

The Transition from Stage Three to Stage Four

In Stage Four, you go back over your life to identify the symbols, stepping stones, memories, and events that stand out as markers along your life journey.

The transition begins with a serious life review.

Where have I come from? If I look at my spiritual journey as it has unfolded so far, what can and does it teach me? Are there any crossroads along the way, where I left certain dreams, goals and wishes behind? Where did I make a commitment to one path and therefore close other options? Is there any unfinished business from my childhood or marriage or family? Are there any emotional doors I closed prematurely or refused to enter or deal with? Are there parts of me that I labeled irrational and emotional? Were there emotions I chose to ignore that now seem to be bubbling up to the surface and take me by surprise? Am I finding my career less than fulfilling? Am I unsure if I really chose what I wanted, or that I went along with the pressure of my peers and family in seeking status, money and their approval rather than going with my dreams and genuine desires? Am I re-evaluating my marriage? Am I married to the partner I really love? Do I want to spend the next 50 years with this partner or have I compromised myself due to my fears of change and losing possibly half of my savings and retirement if I get divorced? Am I prepared to deal with old hurts and anger stuffed away and ignored for years in the marriage? Or have I been single and divorced and afraid to try again and possibly fail at a relationship or just not be willing to make the psychological changes necessary in me to be a good partner? Do I want to give love another chance?

The Stage Four shift starts for many people as early as 30 and continues through the 50s and even the 60s. You are confronting your future from a new vantage point. As you look back over all the years you've lived, you realize you need a new framework. You need a new direction for the true you.

Meredith came to a turning point in her marriage. Her two daughters were out of the home and she and her husband were skirting major issues. He was unwilling to address their differences, so they avoided each other. She was resigned to the idea that they weren't going to be able to communicate and make the necessary changes to continue their relationship.

At that impasse, Meredith began an affair with a married man going through divorce. At first her spirits soared as she began to play and feel romantic stirrings again; she even had the hope that the two of them could be together in the future. She began asking for a divorce, but her spouse resisted. At the same time, her husband went into a huge financial crisis where he lost most of the family money. Finally, when Meredith left the marriage, she had no assets and carried half the debt and half the bills still owed. Add all of this to her gentleman friend's decision not to go forward with his divorce—she felt left out in the cold. It took many years for Meredith to forgive herself, first from some of the poor decisions she made financially and second because of her guilt about the affair. At this low point, she moved in with a friend and literally started over from scratch.

The next few years were spent in therapy reviewing her past, getting rid of the guilt for breaking up her marriage, and coping with the mid-life transition which was the end of her old life with no clear picture of what a new life might look like. She was a single woman totally responsible for herself. The old structures of family, friends and lifestyle were gone with nothing to replace them. During those years of transition, she incorporated her computer skills and began working as a consultant to businesses and corporations. She then began going to workshops, which gave birth to her feminine self. When she realized how important it was to get in touch with her femininity, she reached out to a whole new set of women friends who came to her aid not only emotionally but financially as well. She also worked to develop a financial portfolio, cleaning up the debt and opening new channels of financial supply.

Many questions arise in Stage Four that don't have easy answers. At times, it feels like you are stuck in quicksand. At other times, you feel like the ground is moving under your feet and you don't know where to stand to find sure footing. You wonder if life is more exciting elsewhere or is passing you by, or you feel irritation over not being able to look as young as you want to.

Popular culture bombards everyone with images of youth, so it isn't uncommon for people to feel that looking younger or thinner would be highly desirable. No matter how much I work out, I

The signs of the shift include feelings of ennui, the suspicion that something about your life is wrong or missing.

Depression is inevitably a result from the attitude that life is over.

can't get back to the way I used to look. Frustration results when efforts to regain lost muscle tone or trim down to a weight once easy to maintain repeatedly fail. A similar process happens with cosmetic treatments or surgeries. Some people begin a long and fruitless quest for the fountain of youth or the perfect body. For most, chasing these endeavors can only be a wasted effort, and those who work hard enough to actually look much younger or thinner are behaving in a somewhat regressive manner. In effect, they are saying with their well-maintained bodies that the best of life has already occurred and that there is nothing more to look forward to. After all, how can anyone go back to a time that's passed? I need a vision of how to go forward.

The Lay of the Land

At this stage of the journey it is important to reassure yourself by reviewing all you learned in Stages One, Two and Three—to remember that you are a learner and that the insecurity you feel is simply a natural part of the process of awakening and responding to change. It is time to understand your doubts and confusion, to accept your clarity and own your wisdom gleaned from past experiences. You may try new lifestyles and do things that you formerly criticized. You may even experience yourself doing things that you judged others for in the past.

You may embrace ideas and beliefs that you once rejected.

During Stage Four, you uncover the parts of yourself that you left back in your childhood and which now seek expression. Your playfulness, spontaneity, emotions, and creativity want to be acknowledged. There may be some judgments about these aspects of your personality not being practical, productive, or rational, however it's important to put these judgments aside to discover new aspects of your personality and give yourself the permission to experiment and behave in new and less conventional ways. The playful, spontaneous child wants to come out; self-discovery, curiosity, learning and experiencing new things, going beyond the tried and the true. You may have hidden your dreams and you now are ready to remember the parts you ignored, claiming and integrating them into a bigger, more expansive experience of yourself.

Heidi was married for many years and was now an empty nester. As she began examining her life, she found that she was eager to experience parts of herself that had been severely suppressed by her family. In fact, she never tried many things because her mother had told her that she had no talent. After much internal work, she dared to take singing lessons despite her mother's admonitions that she couldn't carry a tune. Heidi also began taking piano lessons and spending time in amateur theatre productions. Now, through community theatre, she began to develop friendships and expand her social relationships—she felt a new energy and enthusiasm for life.

"Retiring" the Idea of Retirement

Unlike previous generations, the age 50 is no longer considered "over the hill" and 65 year olds are far from rarities. In today's mid-life transition you can add at least 25 more years of active adult life. Given the advancement in medical treatment, the quality and quantity of food available and the overall healthier life- and work-styles, it isn't unreasonable to project living 50 years beyond the age of 50. If attaining the age of 100 no longer seems impossible, turning 50 truly marks a midpoint.

Historically, when the architects of the current Social Security law drafted that legislation in 1937, few people survived to live 60 years. No one in the United States government or the medical community anticipated that life expectancy would stretch, as it has today, well past the sixth decade. The structure set up in the late 1930s has become a creaking relic of its original intention—and an unexpected concern for the baby boom generation. As the huge post-World War II generation nears the age formerly considered a time of "retirement," the system's difficulties will be compounded by the shear numbers of retirees versus the disproportionate numbers of workers.

Today, those people eligible for retirement are encouraged to leave even though they are able and willing to maintain their jobs. In a culture that extols the virtues of "well deserved" leisure time, good company pensions and social security make it possible for older Americans to comfortably step away from the work force. No longer welcome at the office, retirees spend their days in some form of leisure, playing golf or traveling in a recreational vehicle, all of which creates an initial feeling of freedom. The downside, of course, is the end of a dynamic and purposeful life. A distinction now forms between the first lifetime and the second when the mind opens to the awareness and possibility of having 50 more years of life.

Many people never find their way into life's journey. For instance, the Human Resources Department of a major electronics firm contacted a consulting company to do a workshop. The first speaker talked to the employees about the financial aspects of retirement. It became obvious that applying the word "retirement" to the future assumed elimination of the possibility of moving beyond the entitlement of impending leisure time. One worker after another talked about being compensated for all their

hard work. The idea of continuing to work expressively, creatively, and imaginatively, and manifesting happiness as a result of that work, was alien to them.

Some people never leave Stage One or Stage Two, and it's easy to recognize those who have not done their psychological work. Those older people seem childish, rigid, depressed, or bored. They haven't given themselves the opportunity to express the soul through one of the several major avenues for creative expression. Those who haven't worked Stage Three enter mid-life somewhat cynical and jaded. They feel that the world owes them something. No inspiration exists that enables them to mentally accept the concept of something better.

Such people haven't worked on self-esteem or haven't been able to rid themselves of their poverty scripts. They didn't move past enlightenment through pain. They never knew the experience of having their needs validated or being really listened to. Without self-nurturing and support generated from within, they lacked the strength to go after what life had to offer. The issues that weren't addressed in the first curriculum will inhibit further progress in Stage Four.

You discover that you are evolving.

During this period of change, it's important to deal with your discomfort, anxiety, and fears. Far from being a place of security, the status quo feels more like treading water. The Stage Four feeling resembles enlightenment through pain in some ways, but this time the solution is not to work on building self-confidence—that work has already been done.

As you succeed and master the lessons of each stage of your journey, you realize how impossible it is to stay where you are. Each level generates a dynamic energy that pushes you onward. You cannot stay attached to the lessons of a certain stage—not even the gratification and fun of manifesting what you desired in Stage Three. You are pushed to move to the next stage of the journey.

Stage Four Work

In the impasse between past and future, you realize that you can never take time or your life for granted. Even if statistics show you may have as many as 50 years of life remaining, you know that mortality is real. You may have already experienced the death of your parents, siblings, friends and others around you, or the loss of life from earthquakes, the effects of 9/11, or the impact of war. You no longer assume that you have unlimited time.

You know that time is a gift.

You are conscious of the fact that you aren't going to live forever. An inescapable question develops: "What have I done with my life so far?" Evaluating the degree of satisfaction that exists over what has happened so far then combines with an awareness that others are fading from your life. By extension, the mindfulness that your own time will come intensifies every thought. I'm not going to live forever.

As your awareness heightens, an urgency to manifest a personal destiny is actualized. You begin to seek ways to connect to your inner guidance systems so that you can evaluate who you are and what you've done. Am I happy with the way I've lived? What has been and what should be my principles for formulating, planning and creating my life?

Arlene is an example of someone who has worked through and integrated quite a bit of the first curriculum. Yet, she felt an unusually intense restlessness. She found that she could hardly stand to be in her work environment. After years of creating a life that she thought had been crafted to her exact specifications, she was no longer satisfied with the status quo.

She became antsy and was no longer able to tolerate her old patterns. She began to write and journal. She wanted to travel.

Then came a life-changing turning point in her life. The death of her mother made her keenly aware of the dying process. She felt an urgent need to review her own life and come to terms with the person she still dreamed of becoming. She found she had no patience for settling or compromising. Time became very precious. She knew she wanted to move forward. She no longer needed to stay where she was. The same kind of feedback had no appeal for her any more. She thought she'd been successful. What more was there for her to do? What more could she experience? She wondered: "Is this all there is?"

Facing the Shadow

An integral part of Stage Four is facing your shadow, which means opening the door to an entirely new world of possibility. You are able to discover parts of yourself that you would never encounter if you remained with the same people, doing the same things, having the same expectations.

Confronting your shadow was introduced as a concept by Carl Jung, who described it as occurring at or around 35 which was then considered the middle of life, with 70 the endpoint. Mid-life, according to Jung, was an "afternoon" leading to the twilight time of death. At the center of life, Jung explained, people face the shadow by turning their focus inward rather than outward. No longer interested in facades or social roles, individuals at mid-life instead endeavor to get in touch with their spiritual cores.

This is where you can embrace new experiences and ground-breaking types of feedback.

In the first curriculum, family, culture, and education most likely forged your roles and goals. The life review, in contrast, is proactive and generated by energies from within. The vision that results is an expansion of life beyond what was fabricated by the instrumental people in your early years. We go within to discover who we are. The life review brings a larger, more expansive experience of self.

Jeff said that when he was young he played the guitar—but did so only for himself. He said that he wasn't really a performer but, at age 40, he "came out," so to speak. Now he finds himself performing at different public events. For his friend's wedding he wrote a song and performed it in front of 300 people. This was really a stretch for him because it was not something he'd ever done before. In fact, just about a year earlier he had started taking tap-dancing lessons. Jeff noted that his parents did not encourage anything that was related to the arts while he was growing up. They thought it fine to take music, but they wanted him to work for a large corporation after graduation because it was there that he would have security. He had lived a certain way, fit in with the peer pressure, and did the established role. Once he started doing his personal work, he realized that he hadn't had a clue about his heart's goal or what his heart's desire was when he was younger.

The shadow is whatever part you have dormant inside of you.

In the second curriculum, through acknowledging and integrating the shadow, you enlarge your sense of self. You develop parts of the personality that have been dormant, unappreciated, or invalidated. You awaken them in order to expand what you know about yourself. Pieces of your personalities may have been repressed for any number of reasons. They may not have been supported by the roles you wound up fulfilling or the goals you set for yourself. They may have received little to no encouragement from family or society, or not developed because you became successful in other areas. There are many people who may have judged the shadow parts as less than practical. Those parts of self need to be lived out because they haven't had their chance to be exercised or enjoyed.

The impetus for discovering this "shadow" personality comes from within, and the signs are unmistakable. Exceptions to this scenario, in the old structure, were those individuals who were entrepreneurial and creative and who were not dependent on established structure. They approached life in a proactive manner, and functioned without over-reliance on outside validation.

A woman, who has followed the path of being a mother in a traditional family, may need to live out the part of her that isn't a caretaker. She may find herself behaving more independently and learning to make herself the center of attention. Someone in the business world, on the other hand, may need to develop the attributes of nurturing and spending time in intimacy.

Today, people have a harder time trying to live the old paradigm.

Creating a life capable of carrying you forward in a new direction requires being proactive. The usual choice is either working within your existing community or attracting a new group with a vision that is not dependent on former ideas of what behavior is allowed and what is discouraged. When you feel stuck and unable to move forward with passion and vision, you need to recapitulate the past and find the roads that haven't been taken. It helps to recognize the importance of reviewing your life now during mid-life rather than waiting till the end of your physical life.

It is as if you are about to take a running jump—you know you need to step back in order to gain momentum. A similar thing happens when looking forward into the future. Looking back through a life review helps you find the roads not taken—those areas left over- or undeveloped and fallow. It would be good to look back at your goal choices and ask yourself: "Did I choose this because it was my heart's desire, or did I do what society and my parents expected?"

To use myths and fairytales as metaphors, Sleeping Beauty rested unchanged in a glass coffin in the middle of the woods for 100 years and the Sleeping Giant in his slumber became part of the landscape. How was the world transformed when these dreamers awakened? Transition offers us a "time-out" from the usual progression of life and its duration depends on the amount of unfinished business that remains and how many areas exist for self-expansion. Closing out the first curriculum work—of giving and accepting forgiveness, taking responsibility for your own needs, learning, healing, and growing—is essential to moving forward.

Finding your internal Sleeping Beauty or the Sleeping Giant takes time.

Determining what to let go of from the first curriculum, and which jewels of your life to take with you into the future makes for a very dynamic, alive period. It won't be that way, however, if you resist change or try to hold on to past behaviors no longer appropriate to your present consciousness. It's important to take time to discover yourself. You need to be alone with your thoughts and feelings. It's okay to be moody and hang out with yourself without a plan. Create a private, sacred space for yourself. If you haven't journaled before, this is an excellent time to begin.

Bill always knew he was a good communicator. He assumed that his strengths were more verbal than written. It wasn't until he was 23 and in Jungian analysis in Zurich that he began to keep a dream journal. He discovered that he was very good at remembering his dreams. Bill found himself writing pages and pages about his inner-world process of those dreams and images. When it came to writing, he held on to an old picture of the fundamentals of writing. Several years later, he discovered Ira Progoff and his Intensive Journal Writing Method, and Bill began writing in dialogue form about his work, his relationships and everything about his life. Bill realized that he wanted to write a book. He no longer felt satisfied communicating to a few people at a time. He wanted to address a larger audience. His first book proposal got such harsh feedback that for three months he couldn't even go into a bookstore. It was so painful, he couldn't imagine going forward—his ego was literally shattered. He continued to tell himself: I am a learner! I can make mistakes and self-correct. My ego is strong. My needs are strong. My desire is strong. It took nine months to have the courage to start a process of working with someone to share his thoughts and give himself the goal again of writing and wanting to publish.

This is a period where all the gains in the earlier stages might bring you back to being a learner. Stage Four makes it impossible to go back to your earlier successes and feel satisfied. You continue to want more. You can't stay where you were. The areas that make you vulnerable, restless or want to reach out for help are those areas that teach you more about yourself. This phase of transition enables you to create a new life plan and sense of purpose for the future.

There will be bumps when you experience not getting it right.

A key element of facing the shadow requires a process called a life review, which consists of a serious examination and reevaluation of your past history. Therefore, facing the shadow entails developing an inner journey of introspection and self-analysis. A life review is when people dismantle or re-evaluate their roles and goals of the first curriculum with the objective of determining which parts of that life will be taken forward into the second curriculum. What is my shadow? What part of me is missing in my present life?

Life Review

At this point, you question everything. You wonder about your marriage. You doubt the wisdom of your career path or job choice. You might experience the incredible vacuum of the empty nest. Those who've had a family truly wind up considering what it means to be alone as a couple once again. Career couples without children, and individuals that have gone as far as possible within their chosen fields, may question their degrees of satisfaction.

Are there still emotional aspects of myself that I've ignored?

Did I do the right thing? Should I have had children after all? What would my life be like if I'd taken that other job, if I had relocated, if I had opened my own business or I'd married someone else?

What is happening is the closing of the first curriculum. When it ends, you wind up with a new perspective. The life review examines how much work we've put into the issues discovered during enlightenment through pain. For some, the prospect of reviewing and revisiting enlightenment through pain is overly daunting. Those too deeply entrenched in avoidance patterns could wind up having an affair, acting out frustrations, staying stuck in dreams of regaining youth, or becoming irresponsible enough to leave a job.

Individuals tend to put themselves into comfortable spaces where strengths come out and their weaknesses can be avoided.

In the first curriculum, it is possible to avoid many painful things, but when the shadow emerges, you are no longer able to push aside unhappy experiences. You aren't able to move forward without healing the past. Issues show up as problems within marriage, frustrations at work, and patterns of dissatisfaction in friendships. These are typical forms for the reappearance of first-family issues. But by this time, much work has already been done on the personal level. By now, you have identified areas of enlightenment through pain, worked on building self-esteem, and learned to be a manifestor.

In Stage Four, to your great surprise, the intense feelings familiar from episodes of enlightenment through pain may re-emerge. Unfinished business has the power to put you right back in Stage One with feelings like: I'm bored stiff. Some days when I'm driving to work I want to just keep going until I reach the ocean. I miss the kids so much that I just sit in their rooms and cry. Where is that guy I used to be in college? How can I continue to be married to this person for 50 more years?

All the issues that haven't been addressed will return in stronger form. After years of marriage, couples who have not done sufficient personal work have created a museum of resentments. They lack intimacy and no longer know how to talk to one another. Returning to Stage One issues of communication, with the aim of altering old patterns, is essential for the marriage to survive.

Some people who have been successful in careers have ignored certain parts of their growth. Now, in order to move forward they need to create a dynamic curriculum, rather than holding on to the familiar patterns of the past. This requires change.

It is often the case that both partners face issues remaining in their history bank. As they let go of the old ways of spending their time within the business world, and their children are no longer the focus of attention, what do they have to talk about? Suddenly, the "couple" relationship becomes the center of life. This becomes the time when they will need to develop the emotional sides of their personalities, get in touch with feelings, and learn how to communicate, especially if they didn't learn how in the first curriculum.

George was a closet alcoholic and smoker. Every night he came home, had dinner, went into the garage with his cigarettes and liquor to wind down, went to bed by nine and rose every morning around four to get ready for the day. His day began with exercise, reading the paper and getting to the office before seven o'clock. On weekends he played golf.

Agnes, his wife, felt very alone. She felt that she was dying emotionally. To compensate for being lonely, she had been an active leader in volunteer groups and had put her time and energies into those organizations and her children.

Now they were at a crossroads—either she was going to start getting honest about her needs and lack of connection with her husband or he was going to have to re-think his lack of intimacy or they would have to separate. Neither of them really wanted to be apart. When they first came together they were deeply in love and had many years of feeling they were the perfect couple and family. But that way of feeling had eroded over time till there was little or no emotional connection for either one of them.

In the process of doing a major review of their lives, they realized that they had always hidden behind their roles and social masks and now those times were in the past. Since Agnes had so much difficulty containing her resentment, she had to learn new communication skills and ways to share her feelings without attacking George. For the first time too, George had to ask himself some tough questions. Why did it feel so unsafe to be intimate? Why was he so rigid in the same obsessive schedule? Did he want to dismantle his defenses and let Agnes in emotionally? Was he going to stay stuck and not want to change?

How much you are willing to stretch is important for a couple at mid-life.

Often, you cannot continue doing the same dance. What you might not know are the new steps. Do you have enough humility to learn something new? Marriage in the second lifetime cannot be a repeat of the first. George and Agnes had so much invested, and still enough goodwill, that they were willing to put in the time and energy to create a new partnership contract for their second curriculum.

Freedom from Others' Expectations

In the second curriculum, your vision of your future does not come from other people telling you what to do. This time, the vision results from the process of facing the shadow aspects of your own personality. Those parts of self that have been unconscious, dormant, or repressed begin to engage the conscious mind. Discovering or remembering those traits expands the experience of self, which moves you toward the fifth stage of this journey—the time of learning mission and purpose and determining who you are going to be in your second lifetime.

The new curriculum of life has the potential for being an extension, a radical departure, or an entirely new restructuring. Whatever it turns out to be, it most likely will not be determined, as the first curriculum was, by upbringing, family expectations, education, or culture.

Moving Beyond the Familiar

Being asked to let go of something familiar will often become an occasion for fear. This change of nature generates more anxiety than it does a sense of normal progression—one tends to dig in rather than accept the signals that it's time to develop a side of the self that has been ignored.

You cannot create a new curriculum if you haven't completed the first.

If earlier issues stay with you, they load you down. They become the emotional equivalent of excessive baggage on a trip or they fill a room enough to block its normal functions. If you're in a box, you can't open up to new options. For many, the "be perfect" scripts have become so entrenched that the thought of starting something new becomes terrifying. I've been doing what I do for so long, how can I even consider starting over?

Self-esteem, for many, seems tightly bound to career choices, so a total life re-evaluation can raise some questions about how much or whether a drastic change should be made. The stockbroker with years of experience, who keeps thinking about opening a bed and breakfast, and the homemaker with teenage children who was suddenly tempted to enroll in architecture school, may find internal as well as external discouragement. Can I become a beginner again? If the thought of trying something new brings more fear of embarrassment than excitement, you may consider revisiting the self-esteem issues of Stage Two.

A gentleman of 78 decides to divorce his marriage partner of 35 years because he wants to experience the sensual, passionate part of himself that cannot find expression with her. A woman administrator in a law firm remembers she had wanted to be a missionary when she was ten and starts on a new path toward ministry work. A 40 year-old woman who had always been fairly conventional in her behavior and thinking has a series of dreams in which she's a prostitute dancing in a burlesque show. She begins to feel a strong, extroverted energy that makes her want to interact more with groups of people. An "A" level tennis player realizes that he can't sleep after a hard game. He gives up competitive singles without regret and signs up for a yoga class.

The world of possibility is never out of reach.

When you develop enough love and self-validation to see yourself as perfect—wherever you are on the journey—that feeling extends not only to your times of mastery but to times of learning as well.

Staying on Course

A significant part of Stage Four is writing a letter of wisdom to a person you deeply care about. This letter is about sharing the wisdom you gleaned from the first lifetime. It contains the hard-won lessons learned that you bring forward as you cross the bridge into your second lifetime. It is your wisdom, what you have personally experienced. It comes from hard work and blood, sweat and tears. In it is a way of saying goodbye to the first lifetime and sharing what you plan to carry forward. The next four letters were written in a letter writing, mid-life transition workshop.

Dearest Lisa and Sonya,

When I look back at my life, what really counted and mattered most was my relationship to you, my two daughters. When I left you at age seven (I was 31 at the time) I left behind my dearest treasures. I didn't realize in that critical moment when I left how much I would regret that decision and how my body would break down with stress. How could I have calculated how much I would suffer at this loss? I had completely dissociated myself from the role of mother—I was too much a child myself. I couldn't imagine taking care of the two of you alone, without a man. Just as I couldn't imagine taking care of you, I couldn't imagine living without a husband to take care of me. So, when given the choice, staying with you and your father, who didn't want me, or going with a new husband, who didn't want you, I chose the new husband. I then suffered incredibly for having chosen as I did. I finally came to the realization that if a man truly loved me, he would accept my children, my own flesh and blood, as well. So I learned the hard way. Never again would I let go of what was most precious, the bond between mother and child, no matter how insecure or financially unstable I thought I was. You must keep that bond at all costs.

Sincerely, Nadia

Dear Joshua,

Change has played a major role in my life. As you well know, we have lived on both sides of the Atlantic. We have lived in the Southeast, Midwest and California. At one time, I judged myself by thinking that I would have been a better father if I had been more stable, stayed in one place, and put down roots. Now, after living that way for so many years, I know this part of me isn't going to change and I now accept who I am rather than try to be something I'm not. I'm writing because I hope this hasn't been a hardship on you, wishing you had a father who had been more stable and didn't change residences every few years. However, son, what I have also come to understand is that you must be true to who you are and that I was never meant to be in one space for very long. My joy in traveling and changing geographical locals gave me enthusiasm, stimulation and excitement for living, which I hope, has positively rubbed off on you. One final thought—it is important to be who you are and not what others want or expect you to be.

Your father, Chris

Dear Jean,

I'm writing to give you some historical understanding of who I am. I was married briefly and then remained single for 28 years. It has been hard for me to be flexible, make compromises, and not have my way. I can see how willful I have been and how much control I needed. I told myself this was necessary to feel safe. It has taken me till now, now that I'm finally confronting my shadow, to honor the deep effects of childhood abuse and to heal from the unthinkable. Now, as I review my life, I see that I needed all this time. I needed to be totally in control of my living space so that I could heal. I believe I am now ready to explore a primary relationship again. I actually think I can do it. Well, at least I am open to learning how to be close to someone. With some help from my friends and, of course, my supportive therapist Ron, I feel there is a possibility to get married and be with someone in a long-term, committed relationship. Sometimes healing may take a long time. So persevere, dear friend, and amazingly one morning you will awake and feel differently about the world. Now, the future becomes a moment in which the past no longer controls you. Never give up, no matter how long it takes to heal your past.

Lovingly, Alexa

Dear Dave,

I'm writing because I want to share with you some of what I have learned. The single most important piece of wisdom I can pass on to you is to be honest whether it hurts or not. Although it may seem trite, it is always better to be honest and uncomfortable now rather than suffer the consequences later. I had been in a two-year relationship before I met your mother. I was engaged to a beautiful, wonderful woman, but 105 days before the wedding I chickened out. I just couldn't go through with the marriage. Needless to say, she cried and raged, but I held my ground. Everyone told me she was perfect and great and I knew this to be true—although down deep in my heart I felt this relationship wasn't for me. I suffered for ten months, feeling incredible guilt and at times almost suicidal. The moment I met your mother, I felt true love. There was never a doubt that your mother was the one for me. I am so grateful that I waited for your mother and that we had you. I thank God that I had been honest and that I was willing to accept the pain of guilt. Remember son, no matter how painful it is and no matter how much you don't want to hurt someone, you must always be honest if you want to have what will genuinely make you happy.

Love, Dad

The Road Ahead

In stage four, you have completed a major life review. You have been embracing your shadow. Many of you may have had to revisit Stage One. For some of you, this might have been the first time you consciously worked your history bank and processed childhood issues with your family. Others of you may have had to revisit Stage Two by finding holes in your self-esteem when confronted by the fear of growing old. Those of you who had skirted Stage Three, earlier in life minimizing or devaluing money, now are concerned about your savings for the future. Then there are those of you that get divorced and basically need to start over financially.

You are moving through the impasse with a deeper and more intimate awareness of who you are.

Recognizing your shadow, and acknowledging your need to embrace and integrate parts you had ignored, devalued or simply were unconscious to in the first lifetime, has been what Stage Four is all about. It was here that you learned to break down the facades and let go of your total identification with the persona, and get connected internally in a more open, honest and complete way.

The ability to manifest what you want becomes more crucial in the second curriculum, especially toward the end of Stage Four when you begin to visualize more completely the new path leading toward a greater sense of mission and purpose. At this point, your movement toward financial independence intensifies. In Stage Four, you move beyond the responsibility lessons of the first curriculum toward generating an income sufficient to support a broader vision than that of personal security.

> *I don't want to just take care of myself. I want to be sure my spouse is taken care of and my family provided for. And beyond that, I'd like to leave something behind to support causes I believe in. I want to be known for making a difference. How can I become a giver? What will be my legacy?*

Now you feel ready to move forward into Stage Five. You are eager to create a mission and to open new doors of opportunity for self-expression. You want to make a difference. You know you will still be here for a significant amount of time. You want something more than a job or career. You need a higher motivation. You want to make a difference and leave something behind that will have your mark on it. You feel stronger and in some ways wiser. This expanded sense of self is ready to stretch its newfound muscles. With all those years ahead of you, you need a plan; you need a mission. For many of you who were stuck when you first entered Stage Four, you are ready to embrace a mission to go forward with renewed courage and zest for life.

The future appears to be wide open and brimming with possibilities.

Affirmations for Stage Four

- I am open and receptive to change.
- I look within for the answers.
- I am much more than I can possibly imagine or consciously know.
- I let go of the status quo.
- I thrive on uncertainty.
- I embrace the unknown.
- I expand my horizons.
- I dare to experiment.

Questions to Contemplate

- As I come to The Impasse, is there any unfinished business from my childhood, marriage, or family that I need to resolve?
- Are there any crossroads along the way where I left certain dreams, goals, and wishes behind?
- What is my shadow? What parts of me are missing in my present life?
- What parts of me have I rejected, ignored or have gone unnoticed?

Stage 5

The Heart of the Journey—Discovering Your Life Purpose & Plan

With more time to live, you begin to wonder about the meaning of life.

In this stage, we cover Shifting from Personality to Soul, From "What's in it for Me?" To "What Serves Us All?" and Your Mission and Making a Positive Difference in the World.

As I reflect on my own life, my purpose in my 20s and 30s was to heal myself when I was in enlightenment through pain—then to heal others who were also in pain. My first call for healing came in Minnesota when Anna, who in her early 30s was crippled with rheumatoid arthritis, came to me to get her dreams interpreted. At this point, I had been in Jungian analysis for three years and I asked my analyst what I should do. She suggested that I go public as a dream counselor and charge a modest fee. My first client, Anna, saw me twice a week for $5 a session. Before long, I had formed a dream circle of ten women who talked about their lives and analyzed their dreams.

This wasn't a job to earn a living—rather it reflected my desire to help, to relieve suffering, and to respond to those in pain. The entire group was unhappy, frustrated, and felt trapped. They didn't have a clue as to how to help themselves. As I assisted them in understanding their dreams, they began a process of healing and growth. It was clear that my purpose was to heal and support growth and that, through my own healing and enlightenment, I was now able to respond to others.

In my 30s, I made the decision to get my doctorate because of a film I saw by Elisabeth Kubler-Ross. It was inspiring to see the honesty of her patients, their lack of pretense, and their authenticity as they exposed their pain and fears. At that moment I knew I was not afraid of intense emotions. Rather, I became and felt more alive and alert with the strong expression of feelings and the honest exposure of the human experience. Knowing that I wouldn't recoil, I wanted to be close to people in pain. Out of the motivation to be connected to those in pain, I chose to leave my job at a Midwestern college in student services and pursued my doctorate in psychology and religion.

Intuitions of self-discovery come up spontaneously in your life journey—these are insights and perceptions of the soul. Sometimes you'll respond and follow through, or you can experience these insights momentarily and then they escape you. They may even be pure moments of mystical happenings or epiphanies that engage you in the here and now. You will know the soul is involved when you want to share or express or communicate or give or reach out to others around you.

When I reached my 40s, I had a thriving counseling practice. You could say I turned my "mission to heal" into a successful and profitable career. I also created a thriving group practice and actualized a therapeutic healing community. When I turned 50, I no longer wanted to continue with the career of being a counselor, so I began dismantling my practice and proceeded to embrace my shadow. I wanted to identify the genuine self beyond my roles. Or, regain the parts of myself I had lost along the path of success.

As I looked back, I realized that I needed a deeper purpose and sense of meaning beyond manifesting my personal goals. I was ready to discover how I could feel more passion in my life. It was time to find the sleeping giant inside of me and create a new mission and purpose. How could I evolve rather than age? How could I be turned on to life rather than recoil from it? How could I contribute? How could I be reborn and sizzle with enthusiasm once again?

It was in that context, when on retreat in Mexico, that I realized I wanted to be an active voice in the spiritual awakening of the planet. I knew I wanted to be a teacher who communicated truth—albeit my truth. My desire was to go beyond the four walls of my consulting room into the larger community to communicate through the written and spoken word, to communicate words that inspire and empower and give meaning to life. This realization gave birth to the writing of the first edition of *The Bridge*, written in 1999.

The Lay of the Land

The first four stages of *The Bridge* are concentrated on the personal self. During Stage One, you are self-centered and preoccupied with your pain and healing, your biography, your parents, your feelings, and your childhood. In Stage Two, you focused on loving yourself, developing a healthy self-esteem, and giving yourself unconditional love, acceptance and self-respect. In Stage Three, you centered on accomplishing your goals and manifesting your desires. You were a creator and manifestor—you achieved. You experienced personal success and happiness, wealth and prestige.

Have you asked yourself—how am I best suited to serve humanity?

Stage Four found you embracing your shadow—integrating the repressed and dormant sides of your personality. It was a time of discovering more about yourself and finding out what you had forgotten, didn't know, or didn't have the time to develop. In the first curriculum, biology and the creation of a family were the main reasons for being here: The propagation of the species, getting your needs met, getting an education, getting a job, getting married, then raising a family—became primary.

In contrast, you know you are entering in or at Stage Five when your focus to make a difference—to create a future that makes a contribution. Erickson coined the phrase "grand generative," which means—what benefits the whole is more important than personal gain and self-aggrandizement. It is therefore important to define what "enough" is for you.

When Eleanor and Harold began to evaluate their role as consumers. In fact, they met with the hard realization that they were preoccupied with being consumers. They had made a lot of money and lived nicely. They sent their children to the best schools. They joined a country club. They traveled extensively. Now, they began to evaluate what they genuinely needed and wanted and whether their consumer lifestyle was still as satisfying as it once had been. Although they had enough money to buy anything they wanted or desired, they felt out of control. They had to work long and hard to maintain that lifestyle and it didn't seem to be as fulfilling or rewarding as it had been in the past. It was at this turning point that they decided to re-evaluate. They began to ask the question "what is enough?" What did they need to make their lives really happy? Did they experience peace of mind? Was this way of living healthy for them? Did they need a new picture of themselves that expanded beyond their personal pleasure and consumption?

This is true for many of you when you reach Stage Five, particularly if you have demonstrated your mastery of the principles in Stage Three. In Stage Five, personal consumption and pleasure are no longer the primary motivation for living. Now it's important that you feel the urgency to expand your horizons and go beyond "what is in it for me" to how can you make a difference.

In the earlier stages, when you cleared out the misunderstandings and old, outmoded ways of thinking, acting and feeling, you developed a new perceptual system. In Stage Five, you enter deeper into the second curriculum. Here you are ready to move forward to create a dynamic life. You enter this stage as the natural consequence of knowing you desire a more fulfilling life. It is here that you define the many experiences you have had in the world. It gives you time to re-think and plan your future—a future planned according to your self-directed principles, purpose and mission.

The Transition from Stage Four to Stage Five

Some of you may have had glimpses of your purpose during the first three stages. You might even be one of the fortunate few that believed your job or career reflected your purpose. Some of you knew early in life what your purpose and reason for being here was about. However, experience says that most of you were so busy living up to expected goals and roles that you had little time to think about the meaning of your life. You were working hard to fulfill the requirements of the first curriculum, to succeed and achieve, all the while getting approval, recognition and validation according to the standards and values of the current culture.

Stage Five is about projecting forward into time, based on a totally new set of criteria. Your interest is not in retreating from the world; instead, it is that of embracing it from a totally different perspective. You may find that it takes some years of life experience and living to let go of the question, "what's in it for me?" What you are looking for now is "how can I serve the whole?"

The soul's heartbeat is "who am I?" I am a person of significance. I can make a difference.

Mike worked hard for a major corporation. He, like most of us, had bought into the system's ethics of working long hours, therefore sacrificing his personal and family time. All this hard work was with the expectation of a significant retirement package. Suddenly, the company downsized and Mike was out of a job. At this critical moment he felt like the bottom had fallen out of his world. He went into a major depression, feeling like a victim of the system. As he began reviewing his life he recognized that he was capable of manifesting another career, that he could go to another company making a lateral move or perhaps become a consultant. This, of course, would put him back exactly where he was before.

So rather than take the first job offer he received, he decided to take three months to do a major life review. Mike wanted to discover his mission and purpose rather than simply work at a job. It was not began embracing his shadow that he set about doing a life review and began expanding his self-concept beyond his persona. During that three-month hiatus, Mike made the decision to enter the non-profit arena and work for an organization whose mission and purpose was that of service—rather than profit. Based on that decision, Mike and his family began to make some lifestyle changes as well. First and foremost, the entire family decided to budget their money differently so that Mike could rejoin the family.

Sierra having successfully worked several different careers discovered a new avenue of creative expression and purpose. She embarked on a career as a writer and began working in a future-oriented organization whose intent was creating leadership for the 3rd millennium. She was incorporating all her skills into a larger vision of service to the community. Due to a divorce eight years prior, she had to make major changes in lifestyle to the point of having to share a home with a friend. Now, with a new unfolding mission to make a difference and her passion for writing, Sierra developed a five-year plan to accomplish her mission.

In Stage Five, you work with the principles of cooperation, collaboration and non-judgment towards those groups whose beliefs systems are different than yours. Differences are part of the process. In Stage Four, you learned to embrace your shadow—the parts you had formerly minimized, criticized or rejected. As those parts were integrated, you developed a more inclusive attitude and broke out of self-imposed limitations.

You welcome dialogue and are not afraid of differences.

Here, you go beyond your personal beliefs and experiences to gain a deeper understanding of the universal laws. *Love your neighbor as yourself. Honesty is the best policy. What you sow you will reap.*

Your intention is to make principle-centered decisions. You stretch your awareness. Now you make decisions, both personal and professional, that ask bigger questions. *How does this decision affect the environment? Does this profit support better wages for workers in the Third World? Do these deadlines make sense if people need time with their families or need personal*

The inner wisdom has known since birth your life's purpose.

time? You are no longer willing to uphold an image if it means sacrificing personal values or adversely affecting others.

In Stage Four, you found that you could no longer look to traditional sources for answers as to how to navigate through mid-life. In Stage Five, you learn that those answers can only be found by contact with your inner guidance system, through which you can discover your unique reason for being here.

When you add passion to your commitment to serve, your mission will be more fulfilling.

What Does Having a Mission Mean?

Mission means to live your life purposefully—to have a defined purpose. Greg Anderson states that you can achieve a higher level of living by following his life-mission formula—which is VISION+ SERVICE x PASSION = MISSION. He further says that molding a vision consists mostly of a series of judgment calls, including:

- Who are the people who have a stake in your future and what is it that they would like to see happen?
- What are the possible indicators of success in your vision for the mission?
- How can your success be measured?
- How would your vision unfold if you continued on your present path without any major changes?
- What societal warning signs are now in place or are predictable that will affect your vision for mission?
- What might you do to alter the course of events? What might be the consequences of your actions?
- What resources do you now possess or can you obtain that will shape your vision for mission?

- ▶ Of all the alternative possible visions for the future, which are more likely to be favorable to your survival, to your success and to your real contribution to the world?

There is a distinction between mission and purpose. In the earlier four stages, your purpose had been primarily focused on self-healing and personal growth. In Stage Five, the focus shifts from self-preoccupation to discovering a service mission that benefits the whole. People who are living out their mission have translated that mission into action—through service.

Up to Stage Four, you may have worn a mask, which was your public image. In order to perform your mission, however, you must act from your genuine self. Your purpose is to identify your unique talents and disclose yourself without fear or embarrassment. You have goals that support open discussion and free expression among your peers.

The power to effect your mission is directly proportional to the depth of work that you have done in the preceding stages. You could be hampered by not being able to manifest financial resources and be tied to making a living rather than living your mission. You could be afraid of exposing yourself if you had now begun integrating your shadow. This may have an affect on you being able to make a difference. Perhaps you had a dream of appearing naked in front of large audience, during which the facade dropped and you felt uncomfortable because you were exposing what's on the inside. You could also be locked into self-esteem issues, tied to a be-perfect script not willing to risk failure or not willing to take risks. Or, you could still be into anger as a mode of reacting to the world and getting what you want.

If you prematurely did a mission, your effectiveness to serve may have been limited.

In fact, the second curriculum is lived from the view of the soul that knows the vision. It also has the energy, vitality, enthusiasm and joy to carry it out. It is as if the soul has been waiting patiently for the first curriculum to be over—patiently waiting in the wings to step on stage and begin the second curriculum.

The soul has the power and strength to express its purpose over a lifetime.

Steve reached a point when his medical career seemed stymied. His vision of being a physician, how he would practice and how he would be financially remunerated, were drastically changed by circumstances—primarily because of managed care and the insurance companies deciding how doctors would be paid. Steve was at a crossroads. He could either feel like a victim of circumstances or expand his vision of what a healer/physician was all about. In the past two years, he had gone beyond the scope of traditional allopathic medicine by getting acupuncture training and certification. Once Steve began incorporating these ancient processes into his practice, he decided to receive training and certification in homeopathy as well.

The bigger question now was whether he was going to leave the traditional model of practice, change the whole tenure of his practice by incorporating more alternative healing modalities, and, more importantly, spend more individualized time with patients. This meant a significant decline in his earning power and he wasn't sure how his wife would respond. Deep inside, his desire and unique talents were as a healer, but the conditions and his own expanded view now supported some major changes in the way he practiced. Steve knew it would take some time to make the shift. After a few years he had made the move completely.

The Soul

The soul has three parts that are interrelated—the heart, the will and the intuition. The heart is related to love—the feeling, emotional center. The will is related to the ability to execute the power center. The intuition, which understands how life works, is called the wisdom center. When these three harmonize together, the heart operates from love, the will from strength and the intuition from wisdom.

In Stage Five, you will see the soul in a different perspective and learn how the soul thinks. The mind of the soul could very well be called the intuitive mind. This should be distinguished from the analytical mind, which generally reflects your personality, scripts and programming you developed in the first curriculum. Often, you have to work hard to undo those erroneous scripts formed in the first lifetime so that you can find your individual expression of wisdom and truth.

Now it is necessary to open your heart center, which is the organ of the soul, so that you can expand your focus to the soul dimension. Here the inner expression of the soul is love, wisdom and your unique gifts, while the outer expression is your ability to serve. When the soul comes on stage it influences your decisions about how you might serve.

This is where you begin to make the shift from *what's in it for me* to *how can I make a contribution that benefits others.* It may take some time before you will be able to distinguish between dialoguing with the personality and/or dialoguing with your soul.

Now the dialogue is about what is your unique contribution to the world.

Dialoguing with your personality is reflected primarily in the first four stages, such as: *How can I relieve this pain? What do I need to learn from my personal history that will help me heal? What is my relationship to my parents and what have I come to learn? How has my biology affected my life? How can I learn to love and respect myself so others can show me respect and love? How can I manifest success personally and in a career financially? How can I fulfill my roles as mother/father and wife/husband?*

Making Contact and Dialoguing with Your Soul

Before you can begin making contact with your soul, you must first accept the possibility that you have intuitive wisdom inside you. Otherwise, you might even consider contacting your soul to be an act of extraordinary faith. Contact is facilitated by a series of questions. First, you ask a question. Then you have to wait in silence for a response. This response may come through as feelings, pictures, spontaneous insights or revelations. It is here that you take the time to check the question's origin in terms of integrity, truthfulness, and inclusiveness. It is also important that you journal and record your feelings, images and ideas that appear during quiet reflection. Remember that the soul doesn't look for quick answers or quick results even though there can be spontaneous flashes of insight and wisdom when reflecting. When the heart and intuition resonate on your question, you will know you are dialoguing with the soul.

When you begin with the end in view, you begin with the heart of the journey, which is what Stage Five is about.

It has been said that getting in touch with the soul begins with the end-of-life in view. It is there that you reflect on such questions that are most important at the end of your life. What do I want to hear about myself at the gravesite during my funeral? Did I love well? Did I live fully? Did I learn to let go?

When you are listening to your soul you will have a feeling of gratitude, peace, serenity, loving kindness and goodwill. The questions you ask might be: How does the soul's wisdom lead you toward service? Do I experience joy in action? How can I serve/ who can I serve? Who am I? What is my unique contribution? How can I make a difference?

Martha knew she was at a crossroads. Up till now she had been working with an agency that helped people get through the grieving process. However, she felt an enormous need to make some changes in her life. The conflict was that she didn't know what those changes might be. Martha also knew that all the answers she was looking for were inside. To actuate this process, she borrowed a friend's mountain cabin. Making sure that no one knew where she was going and that no one would disturb her, she decided to give herself a week of solitary quietness in nature. It was there that she hoped to discover what she needed to change in her life so that she could find her soul's passion. She began by asking a series of questions:

Q—If money and time were not an issue, what would I do?
A—I'd rather be traveling, hiking and living in inspirational places of beauty.

Q—How would that integrate with my current profession?
A—I'll organize and offer inspirational journeys to those who are grieving.

Q—Who are the people and resources needed to support this mission?
A—I'll do research to see if anyone else is doing this type of work or perhaps I can make a strong business case so that my current employer would like to fund this project.

As Martha continued this process her energy and enthusiasm grew. She knew she was in contact with her soul. Instead of going outside for answers, the voice of her soul inspired and motivated her. She knew she would need continual contact with her soul in order to strengthen her resolve to pursue her vision and make it a reality.

Stage Five Work

The soul serves out of abundance, not out of a state of exhaustion.

Every stage of the journey prepares and empowers you toward your mission—your calling. Each stage makes way for the emergence of the soul. Your soul wants to express itself, not as a sacrifice of self, but as an enlargement for a greater purpose. The soul believes that you were born with greatness and that the world needs you. The soul sees life as a gift—as an enormous opportunity to give to others.

When Susanna was in her 20s, she was married and a public high school teacher. One day she was offered the opportunity to travel and work in public TV. Her husband, however, wanted her to be at home and felt teaching was a more stable, secure profession. When he didn't give her the needed support, she conceded and passed up the offer. A decade later, she and her husband were operating a successful retail business. Once again, opportunity knocked. Now she was being asked to do commercials for a business on public TV. As her media exposure rose, she discovered that she didn't really want to continue working in a retail business but wanted to communicate her passion for service in the business sector. To that end, she received an opportunity to write a column about how to serve the customer's needs. Her heart was in communicating a message, not in selling a product. She wanted to serve and raise the consciousness of both consumers and businesses.

Like Susanna, you have the freedom to choose to live out your mission because earning money is no longer the primary drive. This is a time when major changes in lifestyle—downsizing homes, evaluating spending habits, time and expenditures of energy—are examined and re-evaluated. Stage Five is not about self-gratification or self-preoccupation; it is about contacting the soul.

As your vision expands beyond the individual to a global consciousness, you view life through the lens of the whole rather than from the point of the individual. In Stage Seven, you will find that you go beyond the uniqueness of the individual soul to the union of the whole.

The individual is no longer the focus of attention.

Remember Eleanor and Harold? When they examined their lifestyle and values they arrived at the following conclusions. First, they did not need the big house that took an incredible amount of money to run. Second, they didn't need more clothes—shopping was no longer exhilarating. Besides, if they moved to smaller quarters they were going to have to downsize their wardrobes. Third, they wanted to take more time off, which meant they would have to work less, and make less money. This, however, would then allow them to have the time to pursue a deeper purpose for being here. Fourth, when they traveled they wanted to attend seminars and workshops to enhance and expand their life mission. Because they had received so much from life, now they wanted to become contributors.

Tony was a disability counselor and court expert. He had moved up the corporate ladder gaining influence as well as making more money. Then, suddenly, he made the decision to get his Ph.D. in psychology. He wanted to work with his wife in counseling couples who were moving through transition. It took three years for Tony to get his doctorate. Upon completion of his schooling, his current firm went through a major reorganization that changed the tenor of his job considerably. Now, Tony was at a serious crossroad. Should he continue in the old familiar setting with fewer opportunities for growth or advancement, or could he now open up a whole new possibility? For so long, he had worked for someone else—now he wanted to make a major shift and become self-employed. He felt his mission was to help other couples create a dynamic life. For himself, he wanted to create an entirely new lifestyle. Instead of going to an office, he wanted to work out of his home. Instead of being given clients, he now was networking and building his own community. Tony's future was full of promise and anticipation.

Your mission could be to communicate these principles to others—by sharing your good fortune and understanding with them—ultimately manifesting not only for your personal good, but to manifest for the good of the group—humanity.

Stage Five is about the soul's vision of how to serve. Service, not as a job or a career, is about giving yourself to helping others and contributing to the environment, the world at large. Now you spend time looking at the needs of the whole. What is the soul's vision? What is the soul's expression? What is the soul's passion? What is my contribution to the whole? How might my talents best serve in the areas of government/politics, education, arts, science, philosophy and religion, communication, and economics.

Staying on Course

You have made the shift into the heart of the journey; the soul is awake and well. You feel your passion bubbling. Each day you enter the meditative silence to ask, how may I serve today? How may you express your unique talents to be of benefit to those you touch and encounter? You wait in the silence and, when you hear that inner voice, it is your intuition revealing the wisdom and guidance that you need to move forward with excitement and clarity.

Each day you choose to make that heart connection, feeling the love within you, opening your heart to attract the people, circumstances and events that will synchronize your efforts to live out your mission. You begin to notice that, as your love intensifies, you attract people like yourself who want to serve and make a difference. You feel a synergistic affect from gathering to you people of like mind whose intention is to respond to the needs of the whole. Later, in Stage Seven, you will be forming your soul groups to enhance that global vision. For now, you are focused on your specific contribution to the whole.

Daily you take time for this contact with your soul.

In the second curriculum, you re-evaluate your friends and the way you spend your time. You evaluate the best use of your energies. You want to have truly life-enhancing and life-enriching experiences. You may even consider moving to another part of the country. Your mission defines where you live and where you can be of most benefit.

Each day you awake knowing what your soul wants to express.

At this time you want to have not only a personal mission statement, you might want a joint mission with your partner. As a couple, you may have created a biological family together during the first lifetime—now you might want to create a psychological, spiritual, global family. Many of the nurturing attributes of parents that you expressed in your biological family can be transferred to a larger family. This is where you combine your joint talents and make a difference together. It can be very exciting for a couple to bring together their expertise from different disciplines and focus on a joint creative effort to educate, to inspire and to heal.

Staying on course means diligently and persistently organizing your finances so that you have greater mobility and freedom to serve. You also feel renewed vigor to make the appropriate choices about your health. You know you have a purpose and an important reason for being here, therefore you want to be healthy, vigorous and strong. You express the magnetism and vital, life-giving energies from a heart that is open and pumping new life, enthusiasm and joy for being alive and making a difference.

Affirmations for Stage Five

- I was born to make a difference.
- I have a mission and a purpose.
- I love to serve
- I have special and unique talents.
- I trust my intuition.
- Within me is the wisdom of the ages.
- I know where and how to serve.
- The more I give, the more I receive.
- Giving brings me joy.
- In silence, I contact the wisdom of my soul.
- I love beauty, harmony and grace.
- My soul radiates joy and love.

The Road Ahead

You are ready to enter Stage Six and wake up the philosopher within you. Doing this allows for the discovery of the "Self" that never dies. In Stage Six, you learn how to realize this possibility not as a hope but as a concrete, real and tangible experience.

Just as you begin to feel the passion of your soul and the joy of service, you will mostly likely find yourself also touched by experiences of death—either through confronting a terminal disease or through the actual death of a parent(s), a peer, a close friend or a spouse. This is a wake-up call to your mortality, which brings into view the temporal experience that your body won't be here forever—that nothing is forever.

When you projected forward to the end of life, you gained a better understanding of what was important and how you wanted to be remembered. Here, the impact of death weighs heavily on your soul and you find that you don't have answers to the ultimate questions about death. What happens after death? Was there a life before this life? Is there another life? The death of a parent is symbolic in that you are now the next generation to die. If you don't address these issues you may go into depression. When you are able to go beyond the ego and personality to the soul and intuition, it is possible to meet and embrace a multidimensional reality rather than feel trapped in a purely physical existence on earth.

Questions to Contemplate

- What are my reasons for living?
- What difference does it make that I am here?
- What direction do I need to take in my life right now?
- If time and money weren't a concern, what would I do?

Stage 6

Seeking Answers to Life's Ultimate Questions

When "the little self" looks into the mirror, it sees the cycle of birth and death, self-doubt, separation, fear and shame. When Spirit (the larger Self) looks into the mirror, it sees eternity—that you are timeless, infinite and eternal.

In this stage, we cover Facing Your Mortality, Awakening The Inner Philosopher, Developing Continuity of Consciousness, and Meditation and Lucid Dreaming.

The View From Here

You are one of the lucky ones. You're a survivor, an achiever, a remarkable human being. You have been reasonably successful in your life, and have accomplished much. You've found your way through the challenges and trials of life and faced your shadow, integrating the parts of yourself that were lost while you were busy fulfilling life's first curriculum. You've managed to sort out your relationships, and now have a deep sense of fulfillment in knowing that you were pursuing your life mission and purpose. You have not only built a rewarding career, but you have also established a solid foundation that should carry you into the future quite nicely. You are at peace, and you are fairly satisfied. All is well in your life. Of course, you know you have much left to do, but you know you're moving in the right direction. If this sounds something like your life, then know that you're in for some major changes again! Life will be throwing you some new curves to deal with.

Intimations of Your Mortality

It is nearly inevitable the issue of death creeps into your consciousness. You already have a sense of purpose for your life, but now you find yourself considering the sobering prospect of death. This can be catalyzed in a number of ways. Perhaps you suffered the loss of a loved one, a dear friend, your spouse, one or both of your parents. Or, you may have even assisted someone with the dying process.

You may also become uncomfortably aware of death on a larger scale. This has been the age of mass murders, terrorist attacks, multiple wars, natural disasters, and rising suicide rates. Cancer and heart disease have reached epidemic proportions. Worse, yours is the first generation of people who have lived with the threat of nuclear holocaust. Never before has there existed such a possibility of immediate extinction of life on earth. These factors have hung like a dark cloud over our lives, and yet are rarely spoken of in polite conversation. What's more, in the last 20 years or so, a series of deadly and tenacious diseases have been unleashed on the planet. And all this is exacerbated by the constant, in-your-face media coverage that brings you the inescapable image of death every day. You've seen plenty of war; destruction and human carnage, much of it carried live on television or shown on the internet.

The specter of death has always haunted human history, and has often been perceived as a tragic aspect of life—a misfortune, an accident, a cruel joke played on the human race. Death is reluctantly accepted as inevitable. If you have a religious upbringing, it may have provided you with an explanation of death, but these beliefs seem woefully inadequate when death impinges on your personal life. Explanations and consolations provide little comfort when someone you love is taken unexpectedly by death, or you are suddenly faced with the prospect of your own impending mortality.

There has been, in this culture, a certain unwillingness to consider the questions that death poses. You don't like to think about death, and would do anything to avoid having to face it. You have often stood mute and fearful at the sight of death, sometimes filled with hot, angry tears, sometimes collapsed into bitter grief and resignation. Usually, when death makes its unwelcome appearance, it shows up as senseless and inexplicably cruel. Death takes away the people you love, and ultimately it takes away your own life.

Endings and Death

You probably have experienced some of the "lesser" deaths, such as a painful divorce1 or the abrupt end of an important friendship. You may be one of the millions who have experienced the premature end of a career, forced out of your job due to downsizing or merger/acquisition. The great American dream may have died for you—or God, or the family, or your esteem of authority, your respect for major institutions, or your hope for the future.

You can't help but notice that whole ways of life are changing or coming to an end in this society. The decline of the traditional family structure has been dramatic. You see that, as more people are having fewer children, families are reaching the end of the line. In many cases, no one will be there to carry on the family name, let alone the traditions. Since Americans move every three to four years, there is no such place as "home" any more. You have felt the death of permanence and stability. You may no longer have faith in undying love. You've seen that nationalism, parochialism, hierarchy, and nearly all major institutions are in decay; you have even witnessed the end of communism. Change, upheaval and disturbing trends are perhaps signals of the end of an era, the death of a culture.

The Lay of the Land

In the first curriculum, you probably pay little attention to death. Your focus is on life—being alive in this world, forming relationships, surviving, achieving. You're identified with the world of the material, the five-senses, the experience of the body. You are more interested in material well being, providing safety and security in this lifetime. The last thing you want to think about is death, or not being here. You may feel that you've just been born (or re-born) and have barely awakened to the possibilities and pleasures of this life. You don't want to think about leaving when you've just gotten started.

And yet, entering into the second curriculum you become acutely aware that nothing in this world lasts forever. This can create fear or anxiety. More importantly, this awareness brings up profound questions that begin pressing in on your consciousness.

When you finally die, and look back at your life, will you be happy about the way you've lived? Will you be proud of yourself? Will you feel that you did everything you could do? Will you approve of your actions, your behaviors? Will you have lived up to your own expectations?

While earlier in your life it was possible to avoid the questions raised by death, it is harder to ignore them now. Of course, you could go into denial and obsessively try to stay young, making your physical health the exclusive focus of your life. Or you could opt for the early death of depression, saying to yourself, "What does it matter? I'm going to die anyway." You know that much of the rest of society chooses to essentially ignore death.

Your choosing to read this book indicates that you may already be asking the ultimate questions about life and death. You are part of a generation that has witnessed the death of "authority." You have chosen to not rely on answers from authority figures who tirelessly tell you what to think or believe. You have chosen instead to find your own answers, authentically, from the inside. You want to know for yourself. And, at this point in your life, these questions have taken on a special urgency for you.

Many people experience depression because they live in denial of death, and have no creative or meaningful ways to explore and answer the important questions. Instead of looking death straight in the face, many people ignore it and therefore can't look at life.

Facing the Death of Your Parents

There is nothing quite like the passing of one or both of your parents to bring you face to face with your mortality. When this happens, you are utterly changed. You can never view life in the same way again. Death has thrust its indelible presence into your life, and you are confronted with the fathomless questions it raises. This can be an overwhelming experience, especially if it occurs suddenly or unexpectedly.

So it was for Marge when her mother died without warning, seven days before her 79th birthday. Her aorta burst and she died instantly. It was an inconceivable shock to Marge because her mother seemed so healthy and happy. But now she was gone and there was no time to mourn. Suddenly, Marge and her husband knew that they were totally responsible for caring for her father, who was left behind—blind, stunned and disoriented. They spent the next two and a half weeks together, trying to adjust to this new reality and to life without Mother. Then, after celebrating Father's Day with them, her father became ill. Within two and a half days, he was completely bedridden. He withdrew, stopped eating and rarely wanted to talk. Two and a half weeks later, he was gone. He had willed himself to die.

The awareness of death supports you in making each moment precious.

In the space of a mere 44 days, both her parents left this life. The impact on Marge was profound. She was 52 years old at the time, and had recently been reading about near-death and out-of-body experiences. She felt compelled to find out what happens after death. And now, with the deaths of her parents, she was face to face with her own mortality.

With Marge's mother, death had come like a thief in the night. Six months before, Marge had awakened from a very intense dream in which both she and her mother were on a ledge in a large canyon. Suddenly, her mother spontaneously leaped into the canyon. She wondered why her security-conscious mother would jump off a cliff, while she (Marge) clung to the rocks and crawled off the ledge. At the time, Marge thought the dream had to do with needing to let go of her own security props, but now it seemed to prefigure her mother's sudden death.

On the other hand, her father's example also caused her to begin thinking seriously about the art of dying. He consciously made the choice to leave, and he did it in the most natural way, without anything but the most basic physical support. Marge knew that he was giving her a gift, teaching her about what was possible in terms of conscious dying. He was done. He didn't have a reason to be here any more, and he accepted it. Marge wondered if she would ever reach the moment where she would decide, "It's time, and I'm leaving."

Her parents' sudden death forced her to begin a long process of re-evaluating her entire life. She had to look once again at her first curriculum, the contract that she had with her parents. Marge had to see whether she had emotionally grown up and learned the lessons that were given in her first curriculum.

Questions for Facing the Death of Your Parents

When one or both of your parents die, you usually have some inner work to do. Not completing this work could bring you right back to Stage One and enlightenment through pain. Here are some of the most important questions to explore.

- Do you have any unfinished business with either of your parents (resentments, judgments, hurts, withholds)? Are you caught in unresolved struggle?
- Have you been able to forgive your parents? Did they accept and forgive you before their death?
- Have you rewritten your childhood script? Or are your parents still controlling you from beyond the grave (financially, emotionally, etc.)?
- Were you prepared for their death? Surprised?

- Were their affairs in order, or in shambles?
- Did you get a chance to say good-bye? Or did you miss the opportunity when they were alive to reach closure with them? And if they are gone now, how will you say good-bye and complete that relationship?
- Do you harbor feelings of guilt or remorse?
- Are you in conflict with your siblings over your parents' estate? Or are you angry about your inheritance from your parents?
- Are you now afraid of your own death?
- Do you feel less secure in the world now that they are gone?

Interrupted Journeys: the Near-Death Experience

If you are asking questions about death and dying, you are no doubt intrigued by the recent spate of books written by people who claim to have experienced death—and lived to tell about it. Published accounts of these near-death experiences have had an electrifying effect on society.1 Partly due to medical advances in resuscitation technology, as many as 13 million Americans have had such close encounters with death (a 1983 Gallup poll estimated 8 million). In the last few years, the mass media has seemed preoccupied with the subject, with an explosion of best-selling books, talk shows, news features and television specials.

Near death experience is an evolutionary device to bring about a change in a higher mode of consciousness.

You notice that these dramatic accounts reveal a remarkably consistent story—the experience of being suddenly set free from the body and its pain. Maybe it's like entering into a long, dark tunnel and emerging into the Light, encountering loved ones who have previously died, coming into contact with "light beings" (frequently even God), reviewing one's life, and finally being returned to the body—first to heal and then to complete one's life mission. You know that many who have survived such an encounter come back seemingly transformed, touched with a sense of peace, well-being and passion for life that sets them apart from most of the rest of us.

These dazzling accounts of crossing the threshold into death and being returned to life may be disturbing to you, or deeply inspiring. You can't help but speculate about what the near-death experience means. You can't deny that these stories from the other side seem to offer a more convincing scenario than the old religious visions of pearly gates and streets paved with gold. You would like to believe that it's somehow true. In any case, it gives you much to ponder as you begin to consider your own relationship with death.

The lesson of near-death experiences seems to be consistent—stay on earth. Resist the temptation to leave. Focus on life, not death. Complete your work here. Use your power of love and compassion to make this material world—the world of the here and now—the best world it can possibly be.

The near-death experience comes as a powerful message of hope to humanity. Not only does life continue after death, but also in our darkest and most painful moments the light will come to show us the way forward. Will we have the courage to follow where it leads us?

Guidelines for Stage Six

What to Expect

In Stage Six, you are initiating a spiritual quest that will ultimately take you far beyond the superficial explanations and beliefs of your culture. You are embarking on a journey that will completely change your conceptions about yourself.

> **The questions here are about your very identity and the meaning of life, who and what you are, why you're here, where you've come from and where you are going.**

As you live life's first curriculum, focused as it is on the material plane, it is easy to assume that you are your body, your feelings, and your thoughts. This is the level of reality that you know intimately. Anything else seems speculation, or a matter of faith. But, as you enter into the second lifetime, confronted with the inescapable reality of death, you come to question the way you perceive yourself. You want to know the truth. You can no longer be satisfied with what other people say about death or what might come after. Faith is not enough for you. You want a direct experience that proves without a doubt what is actually true.

To a large degree, this is what Stage Six is about. If you choose to do the work of this stage, your very identity will be expanded and transformed. During this stage, you desire to know what happens after death and how this relates to your life. You desire to experience the Self beyond the body and the physical plane.

You are not what you have thought yourself to be. You are much more than a brain in a body. You are more than flesh and bone and blood, more than thoughts and feelings, more than material reality. Deep inside, you already know this. You are beginning the search for

your true self—the Self that never sleeps, the Self that never dies, the Self that lives forever.

Stage Six Work

Expanding the View

If you have done the work, at the point of your physical death you will have already been trained in continuity of consciousness and will be able to maintain that state-of-mind through the death experience—and beyond.

Stage Six is a journey in itself. It asks more of you than any other stage, and calls for a personal transformation so fundamental that you may find the challenge a bit daunting. You begin this stage facing the questions of death and coming to grips with your mortality. In the process, you will completely shift your perspective about life and yourself. You are going to move to an entirely new viewpoint where you will perhaps see for yourself what has been spoken of in sacred texts both ancient and modern.

You may witness yourself shifting from a personality identified with a mortal body on the material plane to an expanded Self that has no limits. You may begin to consider the prospects of immortality, an existence that continues forever. You may discover other people with whom you will share the journey. However, know that making such a dramatic shift is not likely to happen quickly or easily. It is a process that requires an extraordinary level of commitment and discipline. In Stage Six, you are embarking on an adventure in consciousness, a mythic journey of the soul in which you will relentlessly pursue the truth about yourself and about the meaning of life and death.

While Stage Five was more related to the world of action, the work of Stage Six includes opening up to other worlds, other levels of reality. You will be expanding the context in which you have been operating, awakening to new levels of consciousness. This stage is one of exploring, questioning, experimenting and discovering. This is the stage when you will consciously seek to know the Self that never dies, where you will seek to know the universal laws and principles, where you will seek to go beyond the impermanence of this life to the infinite and unlimited.

From one perspective, throughout this stage you will be preparing for, and even designing, your own death and transition into what may lie beyond. More importantly, you will begin integrating into your earthly life what you learn from our exploration of death and its implications.

When your smaller self looks in the mirror, all it sees is a projection of the ego—all the programming, the history, the fear, the lack. The mirror of projection hides the truth. If you could look into the mirror of reality, you would see the Self, with all the beauty, light, love and wisdom that reside within. You would have clarity of vision. You would be completely in the present as present. You would know that you are beyond the physical, beyond feelings and thoughts. You are limitless, never-ending, and infinite in your capacity to create.

Developing Continuity of Consciousness—The Inner Voyage

You may never have had a near-death experience to utterly convince you that your life will continue after physical death. You may not be one of those to have had a spontaneous out-of-body experience that will irrefutably demonstrate that you are more than a body. It's also likely that you have not been prone to profound mystical experiences, or spiritual vision, or other altered states of consciousness. And yet, you now have a deep passion to desire to know about these things for yourself.

You may wonder what you can do to explore these other dimensions, to experience the aspect of yourself that is reportedly without form, without limit. There are many avenues you can explore. If you are merely seeking such experiences, you will probably have them. They can be wonderful, inspiring, fascinating and fun—even transforming. But there is a risk in becoming caught up in "eating the menu" rather than having the whole meal. You could easily become attached to the experience, and miss the real meaning.

If you're identified with your physical vehicle, your body, and you are identified with your thoughts and feelings, then it's very hard to be aware of who you are beyond your thoughts, beyond your feelings, and beyond your physical body.

The core mission of your work in Stage Six—if you choose to accept it—is to develop continuity of consciousness, a continuous awareness that will be at your disposal no matter what dimension of reality you find yourself in. This stage of the spiritual journey presents you with the opportunity to awaken the Mind that never sleeps, the Self that never dies.

Whether or not you pursue this path is strictly a matter of personal choice. Whether you succeed is a matter of will. As a learner, you have the capacity to journey beyond the known into the unknown. Developing continuity of consciousness means setting foot on uncharted territory. This is certainly the road less traveled. You are entering into a realm where few have gone before. You may discover new vistas never experienced by human consciousness.

Next are some of the guideposts that others have marked. You will no doubt have to find your own way, guided mostly by your intuition and inner knowing.

Out-of-Body Experiences

Many a daydreaming young student has unexpectedly found herself floating up over the heads of her classmates, astonished to look down and see her body still sitting at her school desk. People in surgery occasionally report finding themselves peering down at the operating table, witnessing the details of the surgical procedure, able to hear the comments of attending physicians.

Out-of-body experiences demonstrate the capacity of the conscious Self to have experiences and perceptions outside the physical body.

Such moments are known as out-of-body experiences (OBE), characterized by one's consciousness momentarily slipping out of the body, allowing perception of the world from a different vantage point. These spontaneous events are fairly common (estimates indicate that five to ten percent of the population has had at least one OBE) and provide vivid demonstrations that one's consciousness is not necessarily limited to the confines of the physical body.

For many, an unanticipated out-of-body experience is a disorienting revelation that there is more to life than the physical plane. For you, it can be a doorway to a new understanding of yourself. As a developed skill, the out-of-body experience can be a powerful way for you to explore the unknown worlds. If you desire, such exploration can put you in contact with spiritual forces that can help you to develop latent psychic abilities, to learn more about yourself and your world, and to expand your awareness of the universe. Out-of-body experiences can dramatically change your perception of life and death, give you a deep sense of peace, and leave you with the sense that nothing is impossible.

Lucid Dreaming

Dreams, when you remember them, are often strange and enigmatic experiences beyond your control. They just happen.

However, there are moments when something far more unusual happens in dreams. You may have experienced a sense of suddenly waking up within a dream to realize that you are in the dream-state. This experience of becoming conscious that you are dreaming is known as a lucid dream.

Most people awake immediately after such an experience, but it is possible to learn to continue such a dream while remaining fully aware that you are dreaming. In the lucid dream, you have full access to all your senses in the dream environment. You can perceive your dream world and interact with it, almost as you do in your waking life.

If you are conscious in the dream state, is that who you are in your experience after physical death? Or at physical death is there also the possibility that you are brought into another kind of experience?

The ability to dream lucidly at will is not a natural gift. It seems instead to be a potential of the human mind to expand into a dimension beyond the ordinary. While not necessarily easy to learn, there can be significant benefits to lucid dreaming. For instance, becoming conscious in your dreams will assist you in becoming more lucid and conscious in your daily life. You may already realize that you spend much of your time in a kind of foggy haze. Lucid dreaming can also be used to improve your mood or psychological state, and have that state reflected in a more calm and stable physical life. Some people even use lucid dreaming for problem solving, or as a springboard for other altered states of consciousness.

It is possible to learn to transition into sleep consciously, with the intention of learning. Each night, as you go into the lucid dream-state, you are preparing for the final shift of consciousness in this lifetime. Your ability to stay conscious in the dream-state is a mirror of your ability to be conscious after you leave this body.

Altered States of Consciousness

As you know, many people have explored a variety of avenues to achieve non-ordinary states of consciousness: Shamanic journeys, fasting, vision quests, religious rituals and ceremonies, yogic disciplines, retreats in nature, isolation (sensory deprivation) tanks, jogging, dietary supplements, meditation, visualization, sleep deprivation, fire-walking, mountain climbing, hypnosis, guided imagery, psychotropic or psychedelic substances, rock music, breath-work, practicing silence, chanting mantras, shamanic drumming, past-life regression, ropes courses, etc.

Altered states of consciousness can provide glimpses into parts of yourself and the universe that you did not know existed. These intensely personal experiences may be transcendental or even transpersonal, offering new views and perspectives of the fabric of existence. You might delve into the timeless dimensions of consciousness, retrieving visions and insights that will assist you in your daily life. These non-ordinary states of awareness can bring you the inspiration and vision that will foster your creativity. With the larger perspective they provide, altered states can empower you in your service to the world. They can give you a sense of freedom with which to pursue your mission and purpose.

Meditation

One of the most reliable tools you can use to develop continuity of consciousness is the practice of meditation. While there are many forms of meditative practice, they all provide a powerful method of getting to know your inner self and achieving a deep sense of peace and well-being.

If you are in a body and breathing, you are a spiritual being.

You might choose to meditate for a variety of reasons—to relieve stress, to increase your focus and creativity, to relax, or to improve your general health and well-being. Meditation has become one of the most popular alternative therapies, and has proven so effective that it is now used to treat stress and illness in mainstream hospitals and corporate offices throughout the U.S.

But meditation is not just a hot tub for the mind. Meditation helps to develop the awareness and the energy needed to transform ingrained mental habit patterns. It can also open you to expanded states of awareness. Whatever the form, as you move through the journey of Stage Six, meditation teaches you to remain conscious and alert while your body moves into deep relaxation. You learn how to quiet your mind, to override its automatic responses and continuous internal dialogue. With persistence, you develop imperturbable mindfulness. These are important skills in your spiritual journey.

Based on a willingness to witness, meditation is an opportunity to watch your mind, your emotions, your body and your environment—without reacting to what you observe. Practiced with diligence and patience, it will show you the nature of your own mind. Meditation is a gentle and effective way to become acquainted with your own true identity, the Self that never sleeps. In meditation, you can strip away the illusions of the concrete mind and come into direct and intimate contact with the Mind that has no boundary and no separation, the Mind that knows all.

Meditation brings you back home to yourself, and allows you to experience the Self. In meditation, you will learn to distinguish your ordinary mind—your ego and history, the self of projection from your true Self. Your ordinary mind polarizes, indulges, validates and projects outward to create illusion, seeing only the parts but never the whole. The Mind that never sleeps is untouched by change or death, has a pristine awareness, is always awake, has universal knowledge, and is limitless.

In meditation, the grasping and chatter of your ordinary mind ceases. Here, in the silence, you can focus and ask the ultimate questions. You can receive wisdom and understanding. You can know your true nature and experience the light of intuition, the intelligence of the heart. In meditation, you can go beyond the experience of the physical senses into the energy fields of multi-dimensional reality. Telepathic communion becomes possible.

The soul is the window to eternity. Meditation removes the bars across the windows, pulls back the curtains, and allows the light—the pure energy of love and peace—to shine through. Meditation opens the way to the Mind that creates; the Mind that operates behind the ordinary mind; the Mind underlying all existence.

Awakening the Inner Philosopher

As you face the awesome questions that come to you during this stage of your journey, you will become a seeker of wisdom and enlightenment. You will awaken the inner philosopher, the detached observer—the silent witness of the soul.

It is important to remember that you not only have the right to ask the ultimate questions, but you also have the right to discover the answers for yourself. As you work through the issues of Stage Six, you will find that the answers you seek can finally come only from deep within yourself. The truths or beliefs of others can never satisfy you. You may be guided, you may be given many answers, and you may have experiences that mirror your guidance. But you must always come back to your own intuition and inner knowing to discern the truth for yourself.

The journey is a continual expansion of awareness and perspective, an expansion of consciousness. What is waking up inside you is the Self.

Your heart will guide you to the truth you seek. You will recognize it by a feeling of deep resonance, a sense of wonder and awe, an experience of yourself and your whole perspective. In Stage Six, you are leaving behind all the old beliefs that you have inherited or become attached to throughout your life. You are moving beyond what you have been taught, what you thought you learned, and re-examining everything you have thought about the ultimate questions of life and death. You are coming home to your own perspective, your own view.

You may feel a bit reluctant to allow yourself to be the inner philosopher. You might feel unqualified or unprepared. If so, it is perhaps because you are overly identified with the little self, the programmed and scripted ego. In Stage Six, you will undergo a fundamental shift in identity, as you begin to acknowledge that you are indeed integrally connected with the Mind that knows all things, the Mind that never dies.

Contemplating the Questions

Stage Six is a time for deep contemplation. You will want to give yourself ample space to consider the questions that your soul longs to have answered. In this process, however, it is important not to expect immediate answers. You can use silent meditation or journaling to activate a creative, contemplative kind of thinking that will bring depth to your personality and tap into your ability to consider what is truly important and meaningful.

As the inner philosopher, you are in search of more than personal truth. You experience a growing desire to find principles and laws that are universal in nature. You want to know if there is a curriculum that goes beyond your own lifetime, perhaps even an eternal curriculum that is part of an overarching universal design.

Death does not take away the joy, but it does teach the transitory nature of life here. It teaches the principle of impermanence. If you are consciously connected to the larger, immortal Self, then the impermanence is not a source of pain.

Here are some questions and issues you will be pondering as you move through Stage Six. You can use these as seed thoughts to focus your meditation and contemplation.

- Are you just a brain and a body? When your body ceases functioning, will you stop? Is there a part of you that will never die? Is there an after-life? What is death?
- Is death final? Do you live but one life that ends at physical death? What were you before you were born? Were you here before? Could you have lived other lives? Could you be living a succession of many lives, this one but a step in your spiritual evolution? Is it possible to recall your past lives, or even to remember your future? Are birth and death doorways to and from the same realm?
- What is real and lasting? What is only passing, impermanent? To what extent is the world you perceive an illusion, based on false perceptions? How can you know the difference?
- If you can become conscious in the dream-state, is that conscious Self who you are in your experience after physical death? Or, at physical death, are you brought into another kind of consciousness altogether?
- Can anything last forever? What is eternity? Do you have a soul? What is it made of? Where did it come from? Is it transitory or eternal? Is there a difference between your

soul and your spirit? Is there a way to exist forever? Can consciousness truly be continuous, without end?

- Is there a spiritual realm? Is the spiritual realm separate from the physical? Are there spiritual beings that have no physical form? Are there physical beings that have no spiritual aspect? Are you a human being capable of spiritual experience, or a spiritual being having a human experience?
- How were you created—by what, or by whom? If your parents were your biological creators, who is your spiritual creator? Who is the source of the life within you? Do you also have the capacity to create? Can your creations endure forever?
- Just as a family received you at birth, should there not also be a spiritual family that greets you at death? Just as you were received into the loving arms of your mother, and the home of your parents, is there not a spiritual home to which you go when you leave this dimension?

Choosing the Spiritual Path—Opening to the Adventure

The soul is a stepping stone to having an awareness of the Self that has no boundary or form, no uniqueness and no individuality.

You are choosing a spiritual adventure, embarking on an exploration of what has previously been unknown or unattainable to you. In Stage Six, you wish to extend the range of your experience and your thinking, to go beyond your five physical senses. Here, through meditation, lucid dreaming and consciousness expansion, you may begin to exercise your once-dormant psychic and spiritual abilities. You will see that your body is but one of many energy systems that make up your total consciousness.

Your awareness of death will awaken you to your immortality—not "some day," but integrated here, in this life, in the present. Immortality can become a living reality.

Choosing the spiritual path does not mean that you have to adopt some religion or a particular set of spiritual beliefs. Instead, it means that you intend to awaken your consciousness to its full potential. Selecting a spiritual practice will be helpful in awakening you to your Self.

The work of Stage Six requires a level of commitment and discipline that may seem extraordinary to you. No doubt, you have read stories of people who devoted most of their life to this part of the journey. The spiritual journey is often spoken of in myths, and success seems to require heroic qualities.

Sometimes it might strike you that you live your life as if you were staying in a hotel room overnight. You do what you want here, make your mess, knowing that soon you will be checking out, that somebody will be along to clean it up. You don't have to deal with the consequences of what you leave behind. It's not your problem. But if you knew for certain that you were coming back to this Earth hotel lifetime after lifetime, you would feel differently about it. You would realize that this is your home. You would care about what happens to it. This is the kind of lesson that death can teach you.

Staying on Course

Finding and Working with Your Soul Group

At some point in Stage Six, it will become clear that you can no longer think of the spiritual journey as a personal, individual experience. The journey can only be completed with others. This is your soul group. An important part of the work in Stage Six is to draw to you, and connect with, your soul group. This will form a crucible of healing and transformation, as well as a structure to support the rest of your spiritual journey. Your soul group is the community of people with whom you resonate deeply, with whom you will share the spiritual journey in the balance of this life—and perhaps beyond. Together, you share a common vision, hold similar values. You share the same perspective. You have a mutual commitment to healing, growth and transformation—for yourselves and for the planet. You are part of each other's mission and purpose, weaving a tapestry of service to the whole.

You began your first curriculum in the context of your biological family. In the second curriculum you can create a spiritual family with whom to experience it.

Together, you envision what needs to be manifested in the world, and choose to co-create together. You operate together with principles, practices and agreements that go far beyond the normal framework of human interaction. In unity, you are choosing not to be passive bystanders, but instead to directly influence what occurs on

In this second curriculum, you will discover that your mission and purpose can only be accomplished with your soul group.

this planet. You feel a sense of urgency and commitment to being conscious and active co-creators of the future.

Each person in the soul group is essential to everyone else, each of equal value, each bringing in unique qualities and aspects. You are developing a framework of consciousness together, a shared mind. You are becoming, in essence, a school of philosophers, fellow travelers on the spiritual journey, seeking answers to the fundamental questions about life and death.

Together, you will learn to resonate and vibrate with the same level of commitment, equally devoted to each other's growth and healing. Each of you will want to invest resources, time, energy and emotions within the context of the group. You will share the same deep sense of belonging, of being "at home" with each other. This is not a belonging that separates you from the rest of humanity. Instead, you demonstrate tremendous tolerance, compassion and acceptance of differences. There is no competition. Goals are mutually beneficial, not for personal aggrandizement. You are interdependent, functioning as one whole, working together towards the good of all.

Planning Your Transition: The Doorway to Immortality

In the 21st century, the old beliefs in immortality of the soul and eternal life cannot be accepted on faith. They must be learned in our experience through hands-on training.

As you journey through Stage Six, you will see that death—like everything else in life—is not everlasting. Death is but a transition from one state of existence to another. If you learn to love life with all its changes, death need not be feared. It can be a time of joyful celebration, an honoring of the continuing evolution of your soul.

In this stage, you have the opportunity to foster a relationship with the Mind that never dies, to enter into a deep dialogue with the Self. If this seems challenging, consider this sobering possibility: If you don't come to know this Mind in yourself, then you are literally trapped in your body. Death then comes not as a matter of choice, but circumstances—another experience of enlightenment through pain.

You already know that death can be entered into consciously as a process, that it is possible to die with purpose and dignity. Much of the work of Stage Six is about preparing for your own passing. However, with intention, it is also possible to develop such a mastery of consciousness as to be able to choose how and when you will leave the physical plane. This is a quantum leap into designing your transition into the next dimension. This is mastery. This will require connecting with the consciousness that is undying, that is eternally evolving and growing. It will involve learning when it is time to make the transition beyond the physical, and how to intentionally project your consciousness to the next plane of experience.

Throughout the spiritual journey, you are constantly redefining and rediscovering your Self. Here you experience a radical expansion until you begin to identify with the larger Self. This is true transformation, a rearrangement of the patterns by which your consciousness identifies itself.

To be consciously training and preparing for death is not morbid. It signifies that you acknowledge the value and purpose of your life. You want to consciously make an appropriate transition when your purpose here on earth is complete. Preparing for your eventual passing will cause you to carefully consider what kinds of connections you want to create with other people, the legacy of love that you want to leave behind. And it will cause you to choose the quality of consciousness that you want to develop—a consciousness that can take you forward beyond this lifetime.

Death in Community

You've learned that death can be entered into consciously as a process, that you can die with purpose and dignity. Now you can go a quantum leap beyond that, into designing your transition into the next dimension.

While you were born into a family, leaving this life is generally a lonely process. In our society, death has been considered something you can only do alone. People are frequently put in nursing homes until death comes. Often, one's mate passes first.

However, with the soul group, it is possible to experience death not as a solitary process, but in an environment of unconditional love and support. Death in this context can be a beautiful, uplifting transition. Your soul group can truly support the one who is dying—physically, mentally, emotionally and spiritually. Together, you have a clear picture of where this individual's journey will lead, and what will be happening in the transition.

With your soul group, you will not die in the way that people of previous generations have died. This will be a new experience, virtually unprecedented in modern times.

Affirmations for Stage Six

- I am so much more than what I ordinarily know about my world and myself.
- My physical brain does not limit my consciousness.
- I am the Mind that never sleeps.
- I am continuity of consciousness.

- I am the Self that never dies.
- I trust my intuitive understanding to guide me through life and death.

The Road Ahead

In facing your mortality and preparing for your physical death, you have expanded your sense of Self. You know the Mind that never sleeps. Ironically, the work of Stage Six has not only prepared you for the after-life, but it has brought you to an unwavering consciousness and awareness that is now integrated into your earthly life. You are totally present, totally alive, at home and at peace.

For you, the end will never come. You have discovered your immortality. Physical death will be but a shedding of the physical dimension, a release into the multi-dimensional reality that you have glimpsed in your meditation and spiritual practice. You have discovered your true identity, the Self that creates all.

You will soon be crossing the bridge into a realm of experience where energy is infinite and unending, where form is but states of energy and information shaped by conscious intention. In Stage Six, you have discovered and experienced the Self. In Stage Seven, you and the Self and the Universe will become One, inseparable, indistinguishable.

Questions to Contemplate

- What is the source of life within you?
- What do you need to complete in order to be ready to die?
- Do you need to learn mastery over your physical body?
- Do you need eperiences of giving and receiving genuine love and caring before you leave?
- What is the legacy that you want to leave behind on this earth?
- What do you wish to take with you when your physical life is over?
- What do you want to accomplish after physical death?
- Who are the people with whom you wish to share the spiritual journey?
- What spiritual practice have you chosen for yourself?
- Are you integrating your immortality into this earthly life?
- Are you ready to be a co-creator?

End Notes

[1] More than 60 percent of all marriages today will end in divorce.

Stage 7

Coming Home—Union with Source

Wholeness, unity and community characterize existence for you.

In this stage, we cover Awakening Your Global Consciousness, Accessing Your Inner Guidance System, and Attracting Your "Soul Group" for Co-creating In Community.

The View From Here

The seventh stage of the spiritual journey is a state of being, not doing, where you feel no separation from all the levels of existence—physical, emotional, mental and spiritual. You feel connected to all levels of consciousness.

The task of Stage Seven is to dissolve the illusion of the separate self and replace it with a deep sense of interconnectedness. Guided by the activation of your intuition, you move from differentiation to discovering the underlying unity, the ground of all diversity. Here you experience life in the unified consciousness. In various sacred texts this state is known as Samadhi, or Nirvana. This is the death of the separate self, the transcendence of the concrete mind. You live in the realm of the timeless, the spaceless, the infinite, and the eternal. You begin "thinking like a mountain," experiencing yourself as the whole rather than the parts.

At this stage, you finally understand the wondrous natural progression of the spiritual journey—*body transcends matter; mind transcends body; soul transcends mind; spirit transcends soul.* You are at last one with the sunlight. You are light. You are peace. You know the Self that you are. You embody the love and the wisdom of all Creation. You know yourself as Creator, as pure consciousness.

The first six stages are about your individuation process—your soul's personal journey. Now you make a quantum leap. You go beyond the personal and individual to the collective and universal. You desire to return to the Source and seek communion with the whole. Stage Seven is about world vision, the evolution of the whole race of the planet. It is true that in Stage Five you moved out of self absorption. It was also in Stage Five that you turned to service rather than your self-preoccupation with consumerism.

Until now, your focus was on the individual soul and its uniqueness.

Now, in Stage Seven, your view is a world vision and communion with the whole. As humanity is moving to interconnectedness, it recognizes that each person is a part of the evolving universe. This awareness gives hope and direction to the fact that there is a larger purpose for humanity; it fosters the realization that you have only begun and that there is so much more that "we" as a race can become.

The Lay of the Land

So you have arrived. You have reached Stage Seven. You begin to understand how to develop a group intuition, a group intention and a group projection of energy. It is in this context that you begin to accept the concept of soul groups—communities of co-creators who are aligned in their visions. A place where there is a feeling of the familiar, a natural rapport, a commonality in values, a true sense of belonging, a tremendous tolerance, compassion, and accepting and valuing differences. You develop a soul group that takes on a unity that transcends space, time, form or role. You are a "communion of saints," in telepathic communication. You begin to elicit the assistance of Master Beings, those who are advanced in their spiritual evolution.

Soul Groups for Each Stage

In reality, the concept of soul groups has been operating in all seven stages of the spiritual journey. In Stage One it operated as a therapeutic community for healing. Why was the therapeutic healing group successful? It was the recognition that you had gathered together, because of your pain and suffering, to support each other through a process of change and healing. It was through that soul group that you were a mirror for the group as they were mirrors for you. This group became your emotional family of choice—the family you always desired and needed. It was there that you experienced the nurturing and support you missed while growing up and where you reframe your internal history bank by turning pain into enlightenment. You also learned that forgiveness was the key to healing.

The guiding principle of soul groups in Stage One is *healing*.

In Stage Two, the soul group manifested by you created a positive self-image. This was a group experience where you knew it was going to be safe. You surrounded yourself with people who loved and supported you. There you dismantled the "be perfect" script. At that point, you let go of some of your old friends and groups that focused on blaming or being victims. In fact, you chose to be around people who believed that they were deserving of happiness and love. You found yourself mutually supporting more positive, life—affirming scripts.

Stage Three was about manifesting as a team within a company or a business where you worked towards consensus and common goals. This soul group lived the principles of manifestation; it set and achieved its stated goals. Unlike groups in Stages One and Two, this group used mental techniques, whereas groups in the earlier stages found developing emotional techniques to be more important.

The Stage Four soul group was specifically for people at "the bridge" or what is referred to as the mid-life transition. Instead of going into the familiar, the status quo, you stepped into a group where there were differences. The group then became a place where you lived out parts of yourself that could not have been realized before. You found that tremendous support was needed in reference to the empty nest, leaving an old work situation, or questioning the structure of your marriage. Most everyone in this group had to let go of old roles and goals, and has gone through a major life re-evaluation. It was time to explore aspects of the self that had been denied, ignored or unknown. The major focus of this soul group was to embrace the shadow and integrate the personality in a more expansive way. In times of transition, this particular soul group was used as a catalyst to move forward.

The guiding principle of soul groups in Stage Four is *integration.*

Once you moved into Stage Five, you surrounded yourself with a group that was giving birth to the soul dimension of their being. This group was ready to serve and make a difference. They explored their vision and mission. They identified their values, clarified their purpose and relationship to the world. You had values that were shared not as a consumer but as a contributor. You gleaned the wisdom of how to give back to humanity.

The guiding principle of soul groups in Stage Five is service.

In Stage Six, you formed a soul group of philosophers who asked the big questions. What happens after death? What came before birth? Was it possible to connect to a multi-dimensional reality? Was there a Self that never dies? What is the Mind that never sleeps? This group formed a community that searched for answers and developed disciplines and practices for achieving enlightenment and wisdom. No academic degree was necessary; there was a thirst for wisdom, and meaning was essential.

And finally, in Stage Seven, you want to connect with other people who are clear about their mission and purpose, too, and who have reached a level of self-mastery and want to be creators for the future. They desire to create an interdisciplinary collective in which everyone's strengths, skills and wisdom can be integrated into a beneficial planetary vision and plan where all the parts are interconnected and interrelated.

The guiding principle of Stage Seven is *inter-connectedness.*

The Transition from Stage Six to Stage Seven

In Stage Seven, you learn how to access, as a group consciousness, the inner guidance system, the intuition that Deepak Chopra calls the "field of unlimited possibility." In Stage Six, through discipline and the practice of meditation, you learned how to enter what's called "the gap between thoughts." It is the space out of which everything is created through the mind's intention and manifested on the physical plane. It was here that you first experienced the internal "witness."

Now you are going to discover how as a group and community you can access that inner guidance and expand the field of energy collectively—joining energetic fields to create a group or communal planetary vision. Here you are able to access the universal laws and principles for creating your destiny—creating the future.

In Stage Seven, during meditation, you dissolve the separate self and direct your consciousness deeper and deeper into the source of your being—gradually dissolving all identity and sense of individuality through a process of death and rebirth.

It is interesting to note that Stage Six is about death and multi-dimensional reality, whereas in Stage Seven you unravel the notion of a separate identity with the goal of selflessness and freedom. Here you let go of the roles of family, history, and archetypes, accepting the principle of interconnectedness. You find that uniqueness is not a characteristic of any of these later stages in your journey. Instead, up till now you have been looking at the micro, the smallest part.

Stage Seven is where you understand that you do not exist as a separate being—that is an illusion.

You begin to see the macro, the whole. It's as if the wave loses all of its separate definition in the scope of the ocean. The interconnectedness of the whole is more important than the individual parts in Stage Seven.

The remaining gap is the space between your thoughts. For some this gap may be a narrow band, for others it may be larger. It is the place of stillness and silence. The source of all manifestation comes from that gap or point of silence. And, as you learn to enter the gap and feel comfortable, you can decide where you want to go in consciousness—past, past life, forward, present, this reality, or out of body. This is the point of decision where you have the potential to activate yourself as a multi-dimensional being.

The Tibetan Book of the Dead says it best. "When you experience bliss, it is a sign that desire has temporarily dissolved. When you experience real clarity, it's a sign that aggression has temporarily ceased. And when you experience a state of absence of thought, it's a sign that your ignorance has temporarily died."

Staying on Course

Remember all seven stages are "spiritual." You can, however, find yourself back in Stages One, Two or Three at any time depending on circumstances in your life. Those of you who are working primarily in the second curriculum—Stages Four, Five, Six and Seven—will experience a lot of movement between the stages. The second curriculum is not linear even though it expresses a natural unfolding and feels as if it has an internal logic. Stage Seven is therefore the culmination or self-realization of both the first and second curriculums. However, self-realization invokes the principle of interconnectedness, which includes all of humanity, not simply a personal experience—and yet it is both private and collective. Your soul group, the community that carries your collective global vision through intention, is consciously influencing your personal and collective destiny. No aspect of your personal or collective experience is separate from the spiritual. The old secular/sacred dichotomy is replaced with a holistic vision that all of life is spiritual.

Affirmations for Stage Seven

- I am light, there is no time.
- I am love, there is no fear.
- I am life, there is no death.
- I am pure consciousness.
- I am the field of infinite possibilities.
- I am interdependent with all of life.
- I live in a field of pure potentiality.
- I am the Universe. I am a universal consciousness.

The Road Ahead

A Creed for the Third Millennium

- Your life is a spiritual journey, a process of unfolding and evolving over time.
- There are seven distinct stages of the journey, and they can be understood and mastered.
- Your spiritual journey includes the transitions of birth and death.
- Understanding the seven stages of the journey gives you a perspective in which you can see that all of your life is spiritual.
- "Spiritual" isn't something outside your worldly experience; rather it is the perspective from which the meaning and purpose of each stage in your life can be understood.
- Your success and happiness in life is supported and enhanced when you have a view of the whole, when you can see your momentary obligations, demands, crises and misfortunes from this larger perspective.
- Every breath, every action, every second of your life has had a meaning and purpose. It is moving organically towards a goal. Nothing has been in vain.
- There is a plan and a purpose for your life. Your life plan moves you along your life's journey, through the seven stages. You can discover the whole plan.

- Assistance and support are abundantly available throughout your spiritual journey.
- You do not have to die and get a new body to start a new lifetime.
- Growing into your true Self means expanding your self-definition.
- Your growth is accelerated through connecting with others, finding your soul group, and co-creating a future from love rather than fear.

Sharing the Journey with Your Soul Group

It is a sincere hope that, through *The Bridge*, everyone can identify where they are on their life map. All human beings know that they are spiritual and that life is precious, that wherever they are on their journey is valuable and important, and that they can make unique contributions to the whole of humanity.

As we all do our work in each of the seven stages, we are contributing to the evolution of humanity and the uniting of the whole human race behind a common vision and purpose. We all have a unique role. Through our experience and wisdom, we have the opportunity to identify a soul group where you can collaborate and work to support the growth of humanity. No longer are we passive bystanders. Rather, we are active participants and co-creators in the global future.

This can be viewed as the world vision for the race and its evolution from enlightenment through pain to union and communion with the whole. All humanity is interconnected in its transformation. *The Bridge* gives hope that this life is a spiritual journey and that it has a purpose, a direction, and is intrinsically connected.

The Bridge takes you step-by-step, stage-by-stage through the journey. The whole vision of the life journey is revealed and you realize that you are part of the universe. You have hope and vision. You have a direction. You know the meaning of why you are here. *The Bridge* is a psycho-spiritual global vision for the new millennium.

Marilyn's Personal Experience of Stage Seven

"When the heart is open everything is possible."

When the heart is open, healing and transformation are possible. Since the first publication of *The Bridge* in 1999, I have experienced an enormous progression and movement on my spiritual journey.

In 2003, at a major transition point I had a vision of living by the ocean. I could smell the sea air and saw the curtains blowing in the breeze. I was married to a diplomat and we traveled around the world creating circles of peace. When we returned to our home, it was a professional community as well as our personal residence.

Five years after I had this vision, upon ending a marriage of seventeen years, I moved from Scottsdale, Arizona to La Jolla, California. There I met my current husband, Steve Viglione, Founder of The I AM Foundation. Then, in 2008 the Consul General of Sri Lanka invited us to do a book-gifting mission of *The I AM! Affirmation Book* in Sri Lanka. When I met the First Lady of Sri Lanka she endorsed *The I AM! Affirmation Book* in Sinhalese, Tamil, and English and said, "*The children are the architects of a positive future, and reading and self esteem are the building blocks.*"

Thus, the vision I had five years earlier became a reality and since then I have traveled the world. Together we have also done book-gifting missions in Italy, Croatia, Kenya, Mexico, and throughout the United States.

I feel fortunate to be in my Soul group and a world server. My mission is to inspire and empower children and adults worldwide to express their talents and gifts to make a positive difference in the world; to create a global community that supports a positive and sustainable future and builds a world that serves us all.

I am so grateful to all of those along the path who have made a positive impact on me personally and together we are making an incredible difference in the world.

About the Authors

Dr. Marilyn Powers

Dr. Marilyn Powers is Co-Founder of The I AM Foundation. She has her Ph.D. in psychology and religion. She studied psychology at the C. G. Jung Institute in Zurich, Switzerland and at the Gestalt Institute in Cleveland, Ohio. She is a graduate of The High School of Performing Arts and studied dance at the Juilliard School of Music. Marilyn Powers is a visionary leader, author, and speaker. In addition *to The Bridge,* she is the author of *Words of Power: Affirmations for Loving Your Age, Work, & Life*. She is a philanthropist and has traveled throughout the world doing book-gifting missions for children.

She believes that when children discover their value they bring their value to the world. Equally true, she believes that when parents, teachers, and adults discover their value, they bring their value into the family, the classroom, and the community. Philanthropy of the soul is at the heart of her vision. She believes that children are our hope for peace and a positive and sustainable future. As philanthropists and advocates for children, she and her husband Steve travel nationally and across the globe inspiring children and adults to build a world that serves us all. *The Bridge* is a testament to her belief that each life has significance and that each of us has a calling and a purpose. She believes that together we can make a global leap in consciousness.

For more information, visit www.MarilynPowers.com, e-mail marilyn@iamfoundation.org, or call 619.297.7010.

Steve Viglione

Steve Viglione is the Founder and CEO of The I AM Foundation, whose mission is empowering children and adults worldwide through publishing and gifting The Love~Wisdom Series. Since 1998, his vision has led The I AM Foundation to gift and distribute over 1.1 million books around the globe. Steve is the author of *The I AM! Affirmation Book: Discovering The Value of Who You Are*. The book has been endorsed by the First Lady of Sri Lanka who said, *"The children are the architects of a positive future and reading and self-esteem are the building blocks." The I AM! Affirmation Book* helps children discover their value so they can bring their value to the world.

Steve is also the author of *I Am The Earth: Positive Affirmations for Loving Our Planet*, written to support children in being great stewards and caretakers of the earth. Steve's third and fourth books for children in The Love~Wisdom Series are being published in 2011: *I Am Healthy! Affirmations for Health and Well Being* and *The I AM! Affirmation Book for Teens: Empowering Who You Are*.

Steve's love for children and his unwavering commitment to building a positive self-esteem are at the heart of his mission. He is a global visionary who desires that all children throughout the world know their self-worth, that they are part of the global community, and that their talents and gifts are of vital importance to the future of the planet. The Million Books for Kids Campaign, which he established in the year 2000, supports a global community of children aligned with the principles of self-respect and self-love, that knows *"I Am Greatness! I know others are Greatness too. If you ask me about yourself, I will tell you, so are you."* -From *The I AM! Affirmation Book*

For more information, visit www.SteveViglione.com, e-mail steve@iamfoundation.org, or call 619.297.7010.

How to Contact the Authors

Dr. Marilyn Powers and Steve Viglione offer inspirational programs that empower dynamic change to move in new and positive directions. They are available for speaking engagements and to lead seminars to redefine your life and purpose. They work with individuals, couples and corporations as well as youth groups and community service organizations. They offer philanthropic programs that create new avenues of humanitarian service nationally and globally.

For more information or to contact Marilyn or Steve, please visit www.iamfoundation.org, e-mail iam@iamfoundation.org, or contact them directly at 619.297.7010.

The Love~Wisdom Series
Building Life Skills for Life™

The Love~Wisdom Series

The I AM! Affirmation Book: Discovering The Value of Who You Are English/Spanish Edition

By Steve Viglione

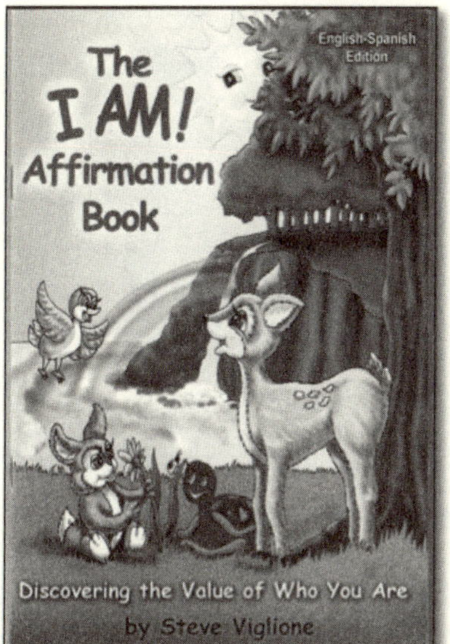

ISBN-13: 978-0-9645224-7-3

Cover Price: $9.95

(More languages available in e-book format at www.iamfoundation.org)

This best-selling book has 165,000 copies now in print. World leaders, teachers, parents and children around the globe love *The I AM! Affirmation Book*. It is a proven tool which helps children to build self-esteem by helping them "discover the value of who they are." Children are encouraged to love and believe in themselves, step into their genius and greatness and make a positive contribution to the world.

Available from: The I AM Foundation at www.iamfoundation.org or 619.297.7010, Amazon.com, & all major bookstores.
Distributed by: Devorss & Co.

The Love~Wisdom Series

The I AM! Affirmation Book Curriculum

by Dr. Marilyn Powers with Wendy Garrido

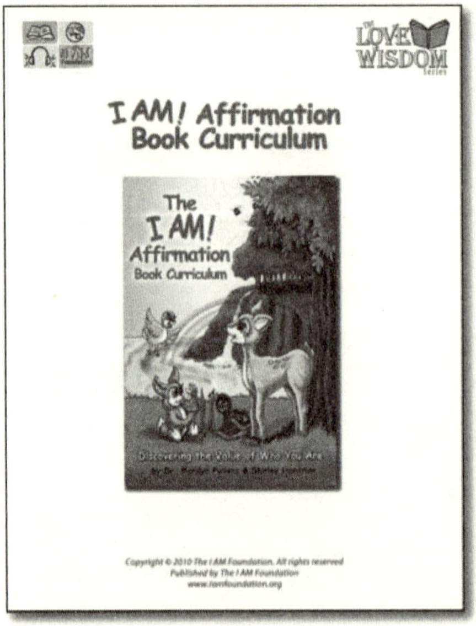

ISBN-13: 978-0-9645224-3-5
eBook Price: $29.95 Hardcopy Price: $44.95

The I AM! Affirmation Book Curriculum is designed to support teachers and youth directors in the classroom or in youth programs. The curriculum (44 pages) gives tools & examples to teach children how to use affirmations effectively in their lives. There are over 20 pages of exercises and supportive materials. Being utilized in public schools and organizations throughout the world.

Available from The I AM Foundation
www.iamfoundation.org

The Love~Wisdom Series

I Am The Earth
Positive Affirmations for Loving our Planet

by Steve Viglione

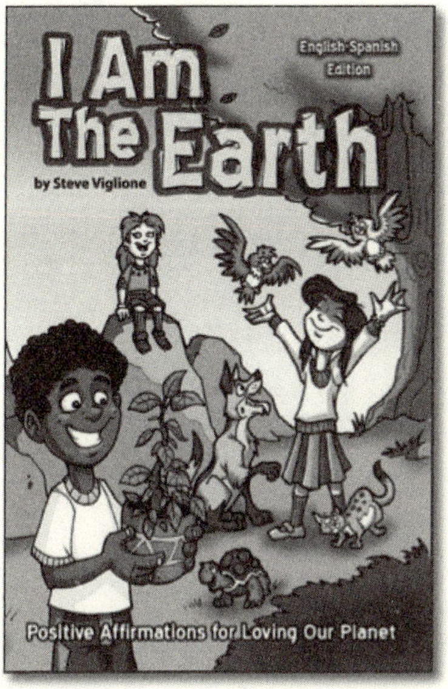

ISBN-13: 978-0-9645224-8-0
Cover Price: $12.00

Support our Planet's Sustainability by ordering the *I AM! The Earth* Book and we will plant a tree for every book sponsored or purchased through The Arbor Day Foundation www.arborday.org. This book empowers kids (and adults) to have an appreciation of Planet Earth and inspires them to use their imagination to create solutions that will preserve and sustain our incredible planet. Our intention is to gift millions of copies of the book and music album to children all over the world so they can connect with how precious and how beautiful this place we call Earth is. We support children and families in being the best stewards and caretakers of the planet they can be.

Available from: The I AM Foundation at www.iamfoundation.org or 619.297.7010, Amazon.com, & all major bookstores.
Distributed by: Devorss & Co.

I Am The Earth Curriculum

Created by Karen Esrtfeld and Roxane Neno

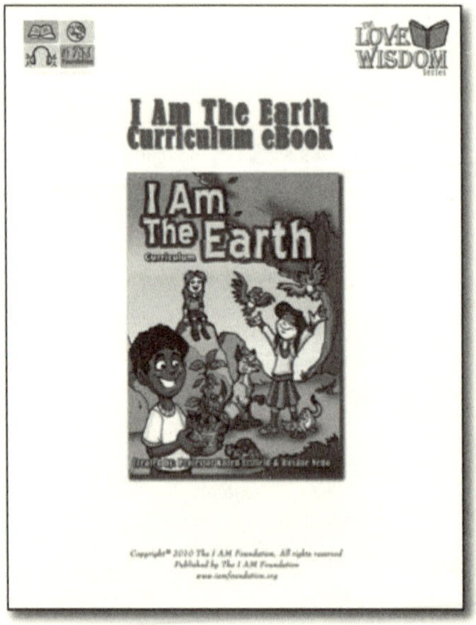

eBook Price: $29.95 Hardcopy Price: $44.95

ISBN-13: 978-0-9645224-9-7

The curriculum empowers teachers and children to discover the wonders of the earth and to engage practically and personally with it. Like the *I Am The Earth* book, it encourages a positive, dynamic and hand's on relationship of admiration and respect between children and their environment. It inspires a desire in children to be great stewards and caretakers of the earth. The rich, in-depth scientific content is extraordinarily helpful for use in teaching. The affirmations are powerful motivators for children to take inspired action for taking care of our planet.

Available from The I AM Foundation
www.iamfoundation.org

The Love~Wisdom Series

Words of Power: Affirmations for Loving Your Age, Work, & Life

by Dr. Marilyn Powers with Steve Viglione

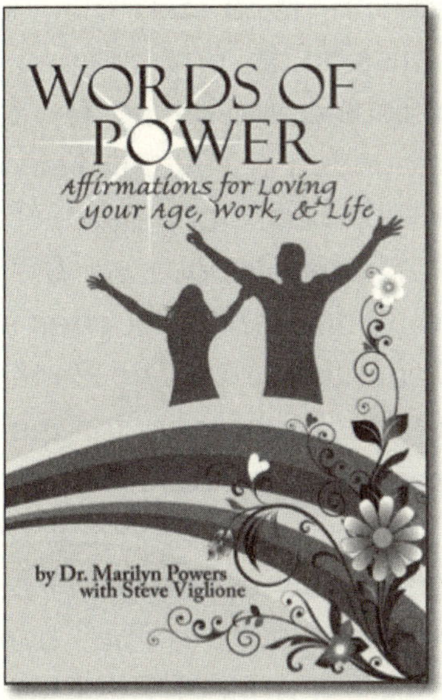

ISBN-13: 978-0-9645224-4-2
Cover Price: $14.95

Words of Power is designed for those who are ready to embrace change, and affirm enthusiastically, "I love my age, I love my work, I love my life!" Love is the most powerful choice you can ever make. When you make the choice for love, you become an irresistible magnet to attract everything you genuinely desire. Love is a gift you give yourself making it possible for you to love your age, work, & life. The choice to love is yours to make. No one can take it from you; no one can give it to you.

About The I AM Foundation

The I AM Foundation is a 501(c)3 educational non-profit organization whose mission is empowering children and adults worldwide through publishing and gifting The Love~Wisdom Series. The organization was founded in 1998 and since then has gifted and distributed over one million books and products worldwide.

The *I AM! Affirmation Book: Discovering The Value of Who You Are* is being translated into 50 different languages and has been gifted in over 50 countries and counting. *I Am The Earth: Positive Affirmations for Loving Our Planet* was published for the 40th Anniversary of Earth Day in 2010. It was featured during Earth Day week on the PR Newswire Billboard in Times Square in New York City. In addition to these books and *Words of Power*, The I AM Foundation is publishing other books for children and adults in The Love~Wisdom Series.

If you feel inspired by the work of The I AM Foundation, you can join us in impacting children and adults across the globe by gifting books from The Love~Wisdom Series, sponsoring book gifting missions in schools and other organizations, or by making tax-deductible contributions.

To purchase books, sponsor a book-gifting mission, make a donation, or to learn more about The I AM Foundation visit www.iamfoundation.org or call 619.297.7010.